Preimplantation Genetic Diagnosis in Clinical Practice

Tarek El-Toukhy • Peter Braude
Editors

Preimplantation Genetic Diagnosis in Clinical Practice

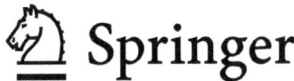 Springer

Editors
Tarek El-Toukhy
Assisted Conception Unit
and PGD Centre
Guy's and St. Thomas' Hospital
NHS Foundation Trust
Guy's Hospital
London
UK

Peter Braude
Division of Women's Health
King's College London
St. Thomas' Hospital
London
UK

ISBN 978-1-4471-2947-9   ISBN 978-1-4471-2948-6   (eBook)
DOI 10.1007/978-1-4471-2948-6
Springer London Heidelberg New York Dordrecht

Library of Congress Control Number: 2013953723

Printed on acid-free paper

Springer is part of Springer Science+Business Media (www.springer.com)

*This book is dedicated to
Ali and Ishrak*

and to

*Professor Sir Robert G.
Edwards (1925-2013),
scientist, mentor and friend,
whose tenacity and foresight
brought joy to so many
through IVF and PGD.*

Contents

Contributors

Gheona Altarescu, MD Preimplantation Genetic Unit, Shaare Zedek Medical Center, Medical Genetics Institute, Jerusalem, Israel

Virginia N. Bolton, MA, PhD Assisted Conception Unit and PGD Centre, Guy's and St. Thomas' Hospital NHS Foundation Trust, London, UK

Peter Braude, MB, BCh, PhD, FRCOG, FMedSci, FSB Division of Women's Health, King's College London, St. Thomas' Hospital, London, UK

Lucie Brown, BSc, Children's Nursing Department of Immunology and Bone Marrow Transplant, Paediatric Nurse Practitioner-Immunology and Bone Marrow Transplant, Great Ormond Street Hospital for Children NHS Foundation Trust, London, UK

Christine E.M. de Die-Smulders, MD, PhD Department of Clinical Genetics, University Hospital Maastricht, Maastricht, The Netherlands

Tarek El-Toukhy, MBBCh, MSc, MD, MRCOG Assisted Conception Unit and PGD Centre, Guy's and St. Thomas' Hospital NHS Foundation Trust, Guy's Hospital, London, UK

Veronica English, BA (Hons) Department of Medical Ethics, British Medical Association, London, UK

Susan J. Fisher, PhD Division of Maternal Fetal Medicine, Department of Obstetrics, Gynecology and Reproductive Sciences, Sandler-Moore Mass Spectrometry Core Facility, University of California San Francisco, The Eli & Edythe Broad Center for Regeneration Medicine and Stem Cell Research, San Francisco, CA, USA

Frances Flinter, MD, FRCP, FRCPCH, MB, BS, DCH Clinical Genetics Department, Guy's and St. Thomas' Hospital NHS Foundation Trust, London, UK

H. Bobby Gaspar, MBBS, MRCP(UK), MRCPCH, PhD Molecular Immunology Unit, Great Ormond Street Hospital and UCL Institute of Child Health, London, UK

Olga Genbacev, PhD Division of Maternal Fetal Medicine, Department of Obstetrics, Gynecology and Reproductive Sciences, University of California San Francisco, The Eli and Edythe Broad Center for Regeneration Medicine and Stem Cell Research, San Francisco, CA, USA

Jan Grace, BSc, MBBS, MRCOG Assisted Conception Unit, Guy's and St. Thomas Hospital NHS Foundation Trust, London, UK

Dusko Ilic, MD, PhD Assisted Conception Unit, Guy's and St. Thomas Hospital NHS Foundation Trust, London, UK

Laureen Jacquet, PhD student Assisted Conception Unit, Guy's and St. Thomas Hospital NHS Foundation Trust, London, UK

Alison Jones, BSc (Hons), MMedSci Assisted Conception Unit, Guy's Hospital, London, UK

Yacoub Khalaf, MBBCh, MSc, MD, FRCOG, MFFP Assisted Conception Unit, Guy's and St. Thomas Hospital NHS Foundation Trust, London, UK

A. Lashwood, MSc, RGN, RSCN, Dip HV Clinical
Genetics Department, Guy's and St. Thomas'
Hospital NHS Foundation Trust, London, UK

Sebastiaan Mastenbroek, PhD Center
for Reproductive Medicine, Academic Medical Center,
University of Amsterdam, Amsterdam,
The Netherlands

Caroline Mackie Ogilvie, BSc, DPhil Cytogenetics
Department, Guy's and St. Thomas' Hospital NHS
Foundation Trust, London, UK

Pamela Renwick, FCRPath, PhD, MSc, BSc
Assisted Conception Unit and PGD Centre,
Guy's and St. Thomas' Hospital NHS Foundation Trust,
London, UK

Sjoerd Repping, PhD Center for Reproductive Medicine,
Academic Medical Center, University of Amsterdam,
Amsterdam, The Netherlands

Genevieve Say, BA (Psychol), GradDipGC Clinical
Genetics Department, Guy's and St. Thomas NHS Trust,
London, UK

Paul N. Scriven, BSc, PhD Medical & Molecular Genetics,
King's College London Medical School, Cytogenetics,
London, UK

Emma Stephenson, PhD Assisted Conception Unit,
Guy's and St. Thomas Hospital NHS Foundation Trust,
London, UK

Fiona Stewart, MB, BS, MA, FRCP, FRCPCH N. Ireland
Regional Genetics Service, Belfast City Hospital,
Belfast, UK

Alan R. Thornhill, PhD Assisted Conception Unit,
Guy's Hospital, London, UK

Willem M.J.A. Verpoest, MD, PhD Department
of Reproductive Medicine and Gynaecology, Universitair
Ziekenhuis Brussel of the Vrije Universiteit Brussel,
Centre for Reproductive Medicine, Brussels, Belgium

Steven Paul Wainwright, BSc, MSc, PhD Department
of Sociology and Communications, Brunel University
London, Middlesex, London, UK

Clare Williams, BSc, MSc, PhD Department of Sociology
and Communications, School of Social Sciences,
Brunel University, Uxbridge, Middlesex, UK

Abbreviations

ACE	Association of Clinical Embryologists
aCGH	Array comparative genomic hybridisation
ADO	Allele dropout
AMH	Anti-Mullerian hormone
ARMS	Amplification refractory mutation systems
ART	Assisted reproductive technology
ASRM	American Society of Reproductive Medicine
AVR	Assured voluntary register
BACs	Bacterial artificial chromosomes
BFS	British Fertility Society
BMI	Body mass index
BWS	Beckwith-Wiedemann syndrome
CBAVD	Congenital absence of the vas deferens
CCT	Certificate of completed training
CF	Cystic fibrosis
CNVs	Copy number variants
CVS	Chorionic villus sampling
DBA	Diamond-Blackfan anaemia
DM1	Myotonic dystrophy type I
EQA	External quality assessment
ESHRE	European Society of Human Reproduction and Embryology
FET	Frozen embryo transfer
FISH	Fluorescence in situ hybridisation
FMR1	Fragile X mental retardation protein 1
FSH	Follicle-stimulating hormone
FSHD	Facioscapulohumeral muscular dystrophy
GMP	Good manufacturing practice

GSTT	Guy's and St Thomas' Hospital NHS Foundation Trust
HCPC	Health and Care Professions Council
HD	Huntington disease
hES	Human embryonic stem cells
HFEA	Human Fertilisation and Embryology Authority
HLA	Human leukocyte antigen
HSCT	Haematopoietic stem cell transplantation
ICM	Inner cell mass
ICSI	Intracytoplasmic sperm injection
iPS	Induced pluripotent stem cell
IVF	In vitro fertilisation
LZD	Long zona dissection
MDA	Multiple displacement amplification
MHC	Major histocompatibility complex
MRCP	Membership of the Royal College of Physicians
MRCPCH	Membership of the Royal College of Paediatrics and Child Health
mtDNA	Mitochondrial DNA
NGS	Next generation sequencing
PB	Polar bodies
PBS	Phosphate-buffered saline
PCOS	Polycystic ovarian syndrome
PCR	Polymerase chain reaction
PGD	Preimplantation genetic diagnosis
PGD-AS	Aneuploidy screening
PGDIS	Preimplantation Genetic Diagnosis International Society
PGH	Preimplantation genetic haplotyping
PGS	Preimplantation genetic screening
PND	Prenatal diagnosis
POF	Premature ovarian failure
PVP	Polyvinylpyrrolidone
PZD	Partial zona dissection
RCOG	Royal College of Obstetricians and Gynaecologists
RCTs	Randomised controlled trials
SBT	Single blastocyst transfer

SCID	Severe combined immunodeficiency syndrome
SMA	Spinal muscular atrophy
SNP	Single nucleotide polymorphism
SOPs	Standard operating procedures
STR	Short tandem repeat
TESE	Testicular sperm extraction
TOP	Termination of pregnancy
TRM	Transplant-related mortality
UPD	Uniparental disomy
WGA	Whole genome amplification
ZP	Zona pellucida

Chapter 1
Introduction

Peter Braude and Tarek El-Toukhy

The Guy's Centre for Preimplantation Genetic Diagnosis (PGD) is the largest and most successful of the HFEA licensed centres that offer PGD in the UK. This book grew out of a number of courses that we ran at Guy's on the understanding, requirements and practical implications of setting up or running a PGD service in the UK. These courses have been attended by a diverse audience: medical practitioners, genetic counsellors, clinical geneticists, laboratory personnel, general gynaecologists, subspecialty trainees in reproductive medicine or fetal medicine, fertility nurses, social scientists and ethicists. We have had much

P. Braude, MB, BCh, PhD, FRCOG, FMedSci, FSB (✉)
Division of Women's Health, King's College London,
St. Thomas' Hospital, Westminster Bridge Road,
London SE1 7EH, UK
e-mail: peter.braude@kcl.ac.uk

T. El-Toukhy, MBBCh, MSc, MD, MRCOG
Assisted Conception Unit and PGD Centre, Guy's and St. Thomas'
Hospital NHS Foundation Trust, 11th Floor, Tower Wing,
Guy's Hospital, Great Maze Pond, London SE1 9RT, UK
e-mail: tarek.el-toukhy@gstt.nhs.uk

T. El-Toukhy, P. Braude (eds.), *Preimplantation Genetic
Diagnosis in Clinical Practice*, DOI 10.1007/978-1-4471-2948-6_1,
© Springer-Verlag London 2014

positive feedback from attendees who have found the information presented helpful to them in understanding this complex multidisciplinary practice. As this information is generally not available other than in large specialist tomes, we have been requested to try and produce it in an easily accessible book.

This book is not intended for the PGD specialist, but rather for generalists who wish to know more about what PGD entails. It is also aimed at those diverse members of a multidisciplinary PGD team for whom some aspects of practice may not be within their usual domain, but who wish to have a deeper understanding of all of the specialist areas involved. For example, the nuances of assisted reproduction and embryology may not be part of the training of a molecular biologist or cytogeneticist; the processes of genetic counselling or molecular testing may be unfamiliar territory to the specialist gynaecologist or assisted conception nurse, but all of whom play a crucial part in delivery of this complex service. It is our intention that the chapters are in language that is easily understandable to anyone who wishes to know more about PGD, how it is practised at the highest standards and what it can be expected to deliver for the individual couple who chooses it as a means to avoid transmission of a genetic disease.

What Is Preimplantation Genetic Diagnosis and Who Requests It?

Most couples planning a pregnancy can do so in the knowledge that they have only a small chance of having a baby with a genetic abnormality. A few, however, are aware that they face a significant chance of conceiving a pregnancy that has inherited a serious genetic abnormality. This may be because one or both of them carry a mutation in a specific gene or because one of them carries a chromosome rearrangement that predisposes them to conceiving a pregnancy with a chromosome deletion or duplication (Chap. 2).

Traditionally prenatal diagnosis has been available in the form of chorionic villus sampling (CVS) or amniocentesis carried out between 11 and 16 weeks of pregnancy. This can be done by chromosomal analysis, molecular testing or in the case of metabolic disorders by enzyme assay. More recently, non-invasive prenatal diagnosis, which can be performed on a blood sample from the mother, has become available for fetal sexing in severe X-linked conditions and for a few other single gene disorders. Whilst some couples will consider prenatal diagnosis and the option of terminating an affected pregnancy, for others this is not the case.

PGD provides the possibility of starting a pregnancy in the knowledge that the child will be free of the genetic disorder. By generating embryos using in vitro fertilisation (IVF), and then sampling a single cell or group of cells from an early preimplantation embryo developing in vitro on which a genetic test is performed, allows only those embryos shown to be free of the genetic disorder to be used to initiate the pregnancy. This may offer a more acceptable way of reducing the risk of having an affected child (Chap. 3).

The concept of preimplantation genetic selection of in vitro-derived embryos is not new. Professor Robert Edwards, Nobel Laureate and one of the pioneers of IVF, had mooted its use clinically following a publication of a proof of principle experiment. In Cambridge, he and Richard Gardner had used Barr body staining to sex rabbit blastocysts developed in vitro. Indeed the first clinical use of PGD in 1990 used sex identification to diagnose and avoid transmission of adrenoleukodystrophy and X-linked mental retardation, both sex-linked disorders.

With the development of genetic probes that allowed identification of specific regions of chromosomes with tagged fluorescent dyes (Chap. 7), and the ability to amplify tiny amounts of DNA reliably using the polymerase chain reaction (PCR), a raft of applications to specific clinically relevant genetic conditions has become available (Chap. 8). PGD now occupies an important place for couples at risk of conceiving pregnancies with conditions where the child is at significant risk of dying early (e.g. spinal muscular atrophy), suffering severe mental or physical disability (e.g. unbalanced chromosome translocations) or having diseases that would manifest during childhood and might, or inevitably, lead to an early death (e.g. cystic fibrosis, Duchenne muscular dystrophy). In some cases, the effect of the genetic aberration is so profound that it results in repeated early miscarriage, later fetal demise or neonatal/infant death (Chap. 2). Many of these conditions are amenable to PGD, provided that the specific chromosomal rearrangement has been identified, the mutation within the relevant gene is known or if the chromosome carrying the specific gene with a mutation can be tracked through the family tree.

Techniques for genetic diagnosis have improved further with the advances in technology, the latest being the use of embryo haplotyping (Chap. 8). This process allows a diagnosis to be made by identifying the chromosome(s) in the embryo that is likely to be carrying the genetic disorder by knowledge of the pattern of closely linked markers in an affected child or other members of the family. The main advantage of haplotyping is that it does not require precise details of the mutation to be known, only which gene is implicated and the pattern of its inheritance in the family. Not only is the development of a disease-specific test faster but also the diagnosis made from a single-cell biopsy more secure. It has superseded also gender selection and exclusion of all the male embryos for couples at risk of having a son affected by a sex-linked disorder, as unaffected males as well as females can be identified easily and considered for transfer.

However with advances in this powerful technology comes increasing responsibility. We need to be aware of public perception of embryo manipulation and misperception of it as designer babies. It behoves us to consider deeply the ethical and social implications of current and future changes in technology (Chap. 15).

PGD Is Not Preimplantation Genetic Screening (PGS)

It has been demonstrated convincingly that there is an age-related decline in the chances of conception following fertility treatment including IVF and an increase in miscarriage. Since the chances of conception can be significantly improved by the use of eggs donated from younger women (Fig. 1.1), it is believed that this age-related decline is associated with a reduction in egg number and egg quality. By not considering for transfer, any embryos that show clear evidence of abnormal chromosomes that are commonly found at miscarriage or associated with clinical anomalies (trisomies 13, 18, 21), it might be hoped that pregnancy rates per IVF cycle could be improved especially for older women or in those patients who suffer

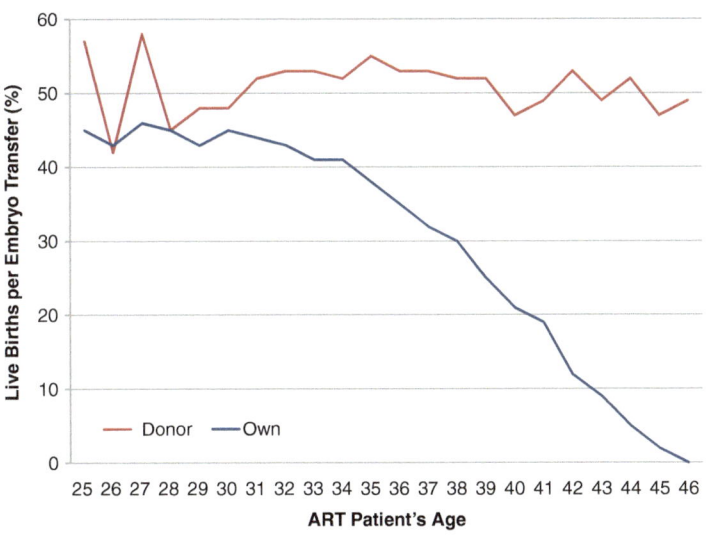

FIGURE. 1.1 Live births per transfer according to age for ART cycles using fresh embryos from own (*blue*) and donor (*red*) eggs (Adapted and redrawn from SART report 2004. Centre for Disease Control Atlanta. ftp://ftp.cdc.gov/pub/publications/art/2004ART508.pdf)

from recurrent pregnancy loss. Detection of these sporadic chromosome abnormalities forms the theoretical basis of the technique of aneuploidy screening (PGD-AS), or preimplantation genetic screening (PGS), which is the most common reason internationally for preimplantation embryo biopsy and is often confused with PGD for inherited genetic disease (Chap. 16).

Is PGD a Fertility Treatment?

Perhaps because of the ubiquitous use of PGS, PGD has erroneously been lumped by service purchasers as just another form of IVF and to be regarded within this domain for competitive funding. Although there may be cases where the genetic anomaly may be associated with infertility such as produced by the azoospermia caused by congenital absence of the vas deferens which accompanies cystic fibrosis mutations, in general the request for PGD is to avoid transmission of the genetic disorder. Thus rather than being allied solely to a reproductive medicine/infertility service, PGD should be viewed as an arm of the genetics service, providing patients with a realistic alternative to prenatal diagnosis and having to consider termination of an affected pregnancy.

How Is PGD Practised?

PGD is a highly demanding specialist technique requiring significant interdisciplinary collaboration. The IVF service and their embryologists skilled in embryo biopsy (Chap. 6) might be regarded in a similar way to a fetal medicine service whereby highly skilled professionals are able to collect a sample of placenta (chorion) or shed fetal skin cells for the purpose of genetic diagnosis. Because of this skilled need, and collaboration between geneticists, genetic counsellors, molecular biologists, cytogeneticists, embryologists and IVF specialist gynaecologists, few units are in a position to offer a holistic and complete service (Chap. 9).

Some units, although having some of the parts needed, may lack the facilities or personnel to undertake embryo biopsy or single-cell genetic diagnosis. In such cases, they may opt to use their genetic and reproductive services for the counselling and initial workup of the patients, but after providing medication and supervising the stimulation of the ovaries to enhance the development of eggs, they allow the egg collection procedure, embryo culture and biopsy and resulting embryo transfer to be done in a specialist PGD unit – referred to as a satellite PGD service.

Alternatively, if the centre has the ability to undertake all the clinical and embryology procedures including the biopsy, they may elect to send the biopsied cell(s) to the specialist single-cell diagnostic unit for the analysis and then undertake the embryo transfer themselves when the result becomes available – transport PGD service.

The majority of units internationally use one of the latter two models, as there are few units able to offer a complete PGD service. As in the USA, the majority of units licensed in the UK by the Human Fertilisation and Embryology Authority (HFEA) (Chap. 17) to carry out PGD use an off-site laboratory to undertake their genetic diagnosis. The Guy's PGD Centre offers a complete PGD service and also accepts PGD patients from two satellite PGD centres in the UK.

Each of the chapters that follow will provide an insight into the interlocking aspects of a PGD service whether practised at a single site or whether satellite or transport PGD is employed. We also explore some of the more complex and controversial areas of PGD, the ethics and social aspects of its practice, future research and development of new technologies as well as training and accreditation. Together they demonstrate the need for interdisciplinary working in order to provide an effective, safe and compassionate genetic service for those who can benefit. We hope you enjoy reading this book.

Further Reading

Braude P, Pickering S, Flinter F, Ogilvie CM. Preimplantation genetic diagnosis. Nat Rev Genet. 2002;3(12):941–55.

Lashwood A. Preimplantation genetic diagnosis to prevent genetic disorders in children. Br J Nurs. 2005;14(2):64–70.

Ogilvie CM, Braude PR, Scriven PN. Preimplantation genetic diagnosis—an overview. J Histochem Cytochem. 2005;53(3):255–60.

Chapter 2
Basic Genetics for PGD

Frances Flinter and Fiona Stewart

Who Requests PGD?

Most couples planning a pregnancy can do so in the knowledge that they have only a small chance of having a baby with a genetic abnormality. A few, however, are aware they face a significant chance of conceiving a pregnancy that has inherited a serious genetic abnormality. This may be because one or both of them carry a spelling mistake (mutation) in a specific gene or because one of them carries a chromosome rearrangement which predisposes them to conceiving a pregnancy with a chromosome deletion or duplication.

Traditionally prenatal diagnosis has been available in the form of chorionic villus sampling or amniocentesis carried out between 11 and 15 weeks. This can be done by chromosomal analysis, molecular testing or in the case of metabolic disorders by enzyme assay. More recently, non-invasive prenatal diagnosis

F. Flinter, MD, FRCP, FRCPCH, MB, BS, DCH (✉)
Clinical Genetics Department, Guy's and St. Thomas Hospital
NHS Foundation Trust, 7th Floor Borough Wing, Guy's Hospital,
Great Maze Pond, London SE1 9RT, UK
e-mail: frances.flinter@gstt.nhs.uk

F. Stewart, MB, BS, MA, FRCP, FRCPCH
N. Ireland Regional Genetics Service, Belfast City Hospital,
Lisburn Road, Belfast, BT9 7AB, UK
e-mail: fiona.stewart@belfasttrust.hscni.net

T. El-Toukhy, P. Braude (eds.), *Preimplantation Genetic Diagnosis in Clinical Practice*, DOI 10.1007/978-1-4471-2948-6_2, © Springer-Verlag London 2014

has become available for fetal sexing in severe X-linked conditions and for a number of other single-gene disorders. Whilst prenatal diagnosis and the option of termination of an affected pregnancy may be considered by some couples, for others this is not the case, and PGD may offer a more acceptable way of reducing the risk of having an affected child.

In some consanguineous communities, there is a high rate of autosomal recessive disorders. Members of the community may have an enhanced level of awareness and come and seek advice about PGD at a very early stage. A few couples may face an increased risk of conceiving a pregnancy that is affected with more than one genetic condition.

In some cases, one partner may be at risk of developing a late-onset genetic disorder such as Huntington's disease. They may not wish to have predictive testing themselves but may wish to avoid having a child who will develop the disorder in later life and so may request PGD. Such cases may pose ethical and social issues, and it is important that these couples have specialist counselling.

Basic Cell Biology

In the nineteenth century, scientists first suspected that the nucleus of cells, which they could see down the microscope, contained the important mechanisms of inheritance. Chromatin can be seen in the nuclei of nondividing cells, and just before cell division, it condenses to form discrete, dark-staining bodies called 'chromosomes'. Humans usually have 23 pairs of chromosomes in each cell (22 pairs of autosomes plus 2 sex chromosomes), and each chromosome contains hundreds of genes, many of which have now been identified. The Austrian monk Gregor Mendel originally worked out the different ways in which single genes are passed down to offspring (hence the term 'Mendelian inheritance'), and his breeding experiments were rediscovered about 100 years ago. We now know that humans have about 30,000–40,000 structural genes, and a mutation in one of these genes can lead to a recognisable genetic disease.

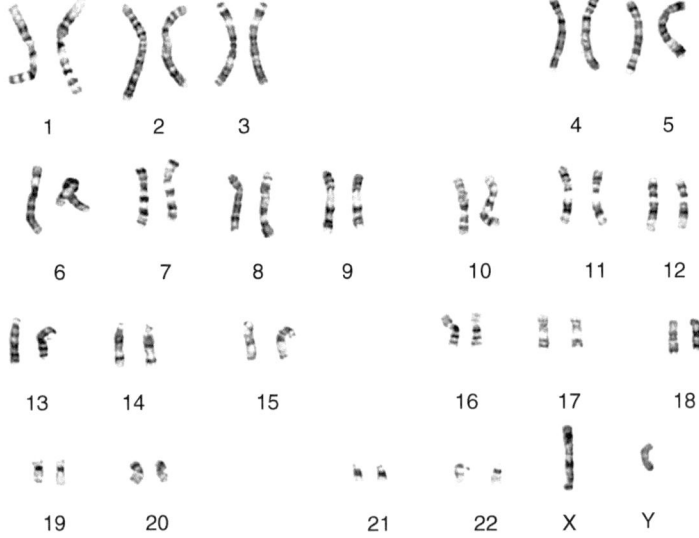

FIGURE. 2.1   Normal male G-banded karyogram: 46.XY

Chromosomes

How Chromosomes Are Passed On

Whilst most human cells contain 23 pairs of chromosomes, the sex cells, or gametes (eggs and sperm), contain 23 single chromosomes, one from each pair. A baby inherits one copy of each pair from each of its parents and consequently a random assortment of 50 % of each parent's genes.

Abnormal Copy Number

Most humans have 2 sex chromosomes (XX for females and XY for males) plus 22 pairs of non-sex chromosomes, known as the autosomes (Fig. 2.1). A few well-recognised genetic conditions are associated with an additional (trisomy) or a missing (monosomy) chromosome (see Table 2.1). Trisomy or

TABLE 2.1 Abnormalities of chromosome copy number which may be viable

Abnormality	Name	Clinical features	Prevalence at birth (female, age 35; female, age 40)
Common autosomal trisomies			
Trisomy 21	Down syndrome	Developmental delay, congenital heart disease	1/338; 1/84
Trisomy 13	Patau syndrome	Multiple congenital abnormalities	1/10,000; 1/2,700
		Severely reduced life expectancy	
Trisomy 18	Edwards syndrome	Multiple congenital abnormalities	1/4,200: 1/1,140
		Severely reduced life expectancy	
Sex chromosome abnormalities			
X	Turner syndrome or monosomy X	Short stature, coarctation of the aorta, severely reduced fertility	1/5,000
XXX	Triple X	Mild learning difficulties, normal fertility	1/2,000: 1/770
XXY	Klinefelters syndrome	Mild learning difficulties, tall, infertile	1/1,650; 1/600
XYY		Mild learning difficulties, tall, normal fertility	1/1,000
Other abnormalities			
69,XXX or 69,XXY	Triploidy	Spontaneous abortion or hydatidiform (or molar) pregnancy	

monosomy of chromosomes other than the sex chromosomes is generally not compatible with survival, but often found in first trimester spontaneous abortions. Chromosome abnormalities occur in 1 in 150 live births and are also found in 50 % of first trimester abortions and 20 % of second trimester spontaneous abortions; however, most of these are 'sporadic' or a consequence of raised maternal age, occurring as a random event rather than being inherited, and unlikely to recur (Table 2.1).

Children with trisomy 13 or 18 usually die in the neonatal period or in infancy. Individuals with Down syndrome rarely have children. Women with Turner syndrome often require donor eggs in order to conceive, unless they are 'mosaic' (i.e. have some cells with normal chromosomes as well as some with a missing X chromosome). Women with triple X usually have children with normal chromosomes, as do men with XYY. Men with Klinefelter may occasionally be able to conceive following aspiration of immature sperm from their testes, followed by intra cytoplasmic sperm injection (ICSI).

Chromosome Duplications, Deletions, Translocations and Other Rearrangements

In addition to the gain or loss of a whole chromosome, parts of chromosomes can be duplicated or lost. A few small duplications and deletions are known to be associated with specific genetic conditions, e.g. di George syndrome (also known as velocardiofacial or Shprintzen syndrome, caused by a microdeletion in chromosome 22). If an affected adult is able to reproduce, they have a 50 % chance of passing the abnormality on to their offspring. Prenatal diagnosis or PGD may be helpful.

The arrangement of portions of chromosomes can also be altered and the resulting chromosome abnormalities may be balanced (no net gain or loss of genetic material) or unbalanced. Carriers of apparently balanced chromosome rearrangements are usually entirely healthy, unless at the site of the chromosome breakage and rearrangement a gene has been disrupted or there is submicroscopic chromosome imbalance. The majority of carriers of balanced rearrangements only find out they are carriers if they are tested as part of the investigation of multiple spontaneous miscarriages, or because they have had a previous child with multiple congenital abnormalities who is found to have an unbalanced chromosome pattern, or because there is a known family history of a chromosome rearrangement. The most common rearrangements are reciprocal (Fig. 2.2) and Robertsonian translocations (Fig. 2.3), found in 1 in 500 and 1 in 1,000 individuals, respectively.

A reciprocal translocation occurs when breaks in two different chromosomes result in material being exchanged between them with the creation of a derivative chromosome. A balanced reciprocal translocation carrier is usually healthy as she/he has a normal complement of genetic material; but their offspring may inherit the balanced translocation, or an unbalanced form, with duplications (partial trisomy) and/or deletions (partial monosomy) of important genetic material. Smaller deletions/duplications may be compatible with survival, but associated with a range of medical problems and learning difficulties, whilst larger chromosome imbalances are more likely to result in a spontaneous abortion.

In Robertsonian translocations the short arms of two different chromosomes are lost and the long arms fuse at the centromere to form a single chromosome. Thus, carriers of Robertsonian translocations have 45 rather than 46 chromosomes, but as no important material has been lost, they are phenotypically normal; however, their offspring may inherit a missing or an extra-long arm of an acrocentric chromosome (13, 14, 15, 21 or 22).

Carriers of balanced chromosome rearrangements often have an unfortunate obstetric history, presenting with multiple early miscarriages or failure to conceive; alternatively they may have previously had a child with unbalanced chromosomes affected with multiple congenital abnormalities. In addition to around a 30 % chance of conceiving an unbalanced pregnancy and miscarrying, they may face a risk of up to 20 % of conceiving an unbalanced pregnancy that is viable

a

A terminal exchange between the long arms of chromosomes 11 and 22 with breakpoints at chromosome bands 11q23.3 and 22q11.2 and no gain or loss of material (balanced).

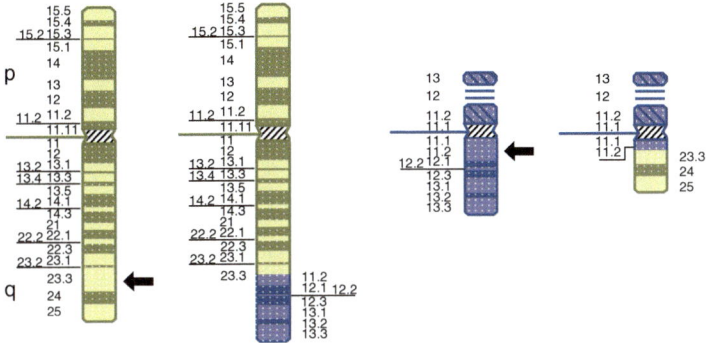

b

Transmission of the chromosome 11, 22 and der(22) in a gamete results in tertiary trisomy for the derivative chromosome 22 after normal fertilization, causing Emanuel syndrome (OMIM #190685), e.g. 47,XY,+der(22)t(11;22)(q23.3;q11.2)mat

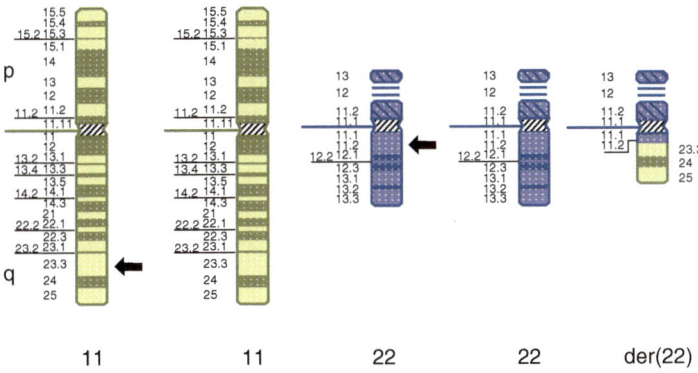

FIGURE. 2.2   Reciprocal translocation: e.g. 46,XX,t(11;22)(q23.3;q11.2). (**a**) A terminal exchange between the long arms of chromosomes 11 and 22 with breakpoints at chromosome bands 11q23.3 and 22q11.2 and no gain or loss of material (balanced). (**b**) Transmission of the chromosome 11, 22 and der(22) in a gamete results in tertiary trisomy for the derivative chromosome 22 after normal fertilisation, causing Emanuel syndrome (OMIM #609029), e.g. 47,XY,+der(22)t(11;22)(q23.3;q11.2)mat

a

Centric fusion of the long arms of chromosomes 14 and 21 and loss of the short arms resulting in 45 chromosomes

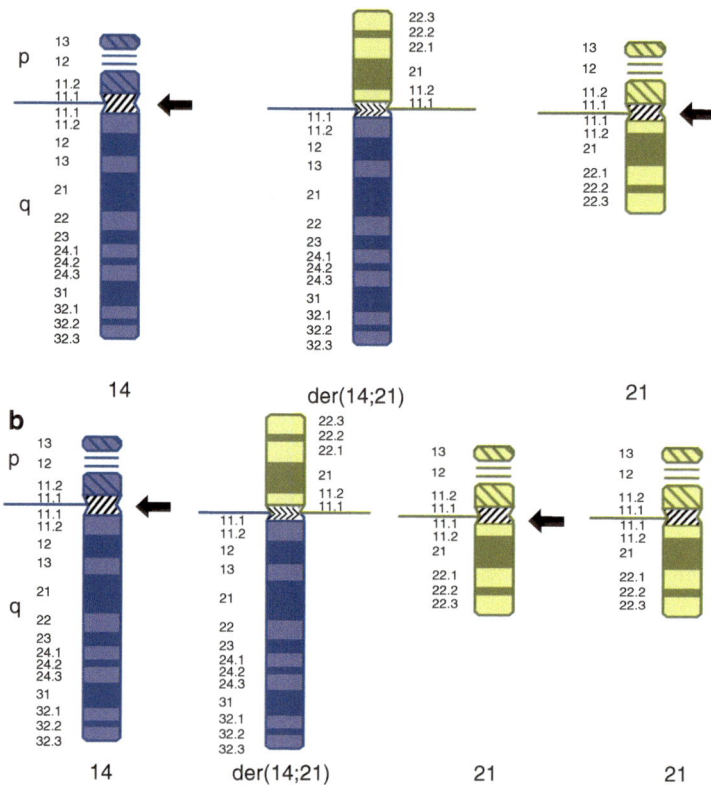

Transmission of the der(14;21) and a chromosome 21 in an egg or sperm results in translocation trisomy 21 after normal fertilisation, causing Down syndrome (OMIM #190685), e.g. 46,XX,der(14;21)(q10;q10)mat,+21

FIGURE. 2.3 Robertsonian translocation: e.g. 45,XX,der(14;21)(q10;q10) (**a**) Centric fusion of the long arms of chromosomes 14 and 21 and loss of the short arms resulting in 45 chromosomes. (**b**) Transmission of the der(14;21) and a chromosome 21 in an egg or sperm results in translocation trisomy 21 after normal fertilisation, causing Down syndrome (OMIM #190685), e.g. 46,XX,der(14;21)(q10;q10)mat,+21

and could continue to term; for them PGD may be particularly helpful. Even if the risk of a viable unbalanced pregnancy that goes to term is very low, PGD may still be considered as there can be a significant physical and emotional burden caused by multiple pregnancies that are doomed to failure.

Genes

Human beings have approximately 30,000–40,000 genes, but these represent less than 2 % of the genome. The remainder is made up of DNA sequences that are predominantly inactive and has been described as 'junk' DNA; however, some of these regions show evolutionary conservation and may play a role in the regulation of gene expression. The distribution of these genes varies greatly between different chromosome regions; the highest gene density is found towards the end of chromosomes (the subtelomeric regions). Gene size is also very variable: small genes may contain only one exon (coding region), whilst others, e.g. dystrophin, the gene involved in X-linked muscular dystrophy, contain 79 exons. Most human genes code for polypeptides such as enzymes, hormones and structural or regulatory proteins.

Mutations in Genes

There are a number of ways in which the functioning of a gene can be impaired. The whole gene may be deleted, or there may be an error in the DNA ranging from a small (point) mutation to a much larger deletion or insertion within the genetic message. Smaller mutations are not necessarily associated with milder disease as even the smallest mutation may effectively stop the transcription of the whole gene. Over the last 20 years or so, laboratories have identified a wide range of mutations in thousands of different genes, and the underlying genetic cause of a number of different conditions has been elucidated. The actual genetic mutation in a particular family may be unique to that family, which may make it hard to identify; however, in some families, it is possible to track the inheritance of the specific chromosome carrying that particular gene without knowing the precise mutation within the DNA, an approach known as a 'linkage study'.

Genetic conditions may be caused by abnormalities in one or more genes. More than 15,000 single-gene disorders have been identified, and there are three main patterns of inheritance, the characteristics of which are summarised in Table 2.2.

Autosomal Dominant Conditions

Autosomal dominant conditions affect 1 in 200 individuals and are caused by a single mutation in one copy of a gene pair; examples include Huntington's disease, adult polycystic kidney disease and myotonic dystrophy. Anyone affected with an autosomal dominant condition carries a mutation in one copy of that particular gene pair (heterozygous) and has a 1 in 2 (50 %) chance of passing on the condition each time they have a child.

One of the difficulties in counselling families with some autosomal dominant conditions, e.g. neurofibromatosis or tuberous sclerosis, is that even within a family, individuals who have the same mutation may present with very different clinical features. The genetic test can only show whether the person carries the gene mutation or not. It usually cannot predict how severely the individual will be affected. This can make reproductive decisions complicated. A parent who is relatively mildly affected with an autosomal dominant condition may find it hard to contemplate prenatal diagnosis and termination of an affected pregnancy. At the same time, there is a risk that the child may be much more severely affected than they are.

Autosomal Recessive

Autosomal recessive conditions are mostly quite rare and occur when both parents, who happen to carry a mutation in the same gene, pass on their mutated copy of the gene to the same child, who is homozygous for the mutated gene,

TABLE 2.2 Characteristics of Mendelian inheritance

Autosomal dominant inheritance

Males and females affected equally

Affected individuals across a number of generations

Onset of symptoms may be delayed until later in life if not apparent at birth

New mutation rate 0–100 %. The new mutation rate tends to be lower in milder conditions that are associated with normal fertility

Affected individuals have a 50 % chance of passing the condition on to their offspring

Autosomal recessive inheritance

Males and females affected equally

Affected individuals may all be in the same generation

Higher risk in consanguineous relationships

Onset of symptoms is often at birth or during childhood

New mutation rate low

Carrier couples have a 25 % chance of having an affected child in each pregnancy

X-linked inheritance

No male to male transmission

Males much more severely affected than female carriers (who are generally asymptomatic)

All the daughters of affected males are obligate carriers

New mutation rate variable, but higher with more severe conditions

Carrier females have a 50 % chance that any son of theirs will be affected and a 50 % chance that any daughter will be a carrier

having no copy of the normal gene. Examples of autosomal recessive conditions include cystic fibrosis, sickle-cell disease and spinal muscular atrophy. With autosomal recessive conditions, affected individuals within the same family who have the same mutations will usually be similarly affected. In consanguineous communities, there can be an increased rate of some autosomal recessive conditions.

Sex-Linked Inheritance

Sex-linked inheritance refers to genes inherited on the X chromosome, of which females have two copies and males only one. Males who inherit a mutation on their single X chromosome are affected with the particular disease involved, whereas females with one mutated copy of the gene are often asymptomatic because of the presence of a second normal copy of the gene. Examples include haemophilia and Duchenne muscular dystrophy.

Gonadal Mosaicism

Gonadal mosaicism refers to the situation where an individual has two populations of cells in the gonads (testes or ovaries), one population of cells containing the usual genetic complement whilst the other contains a DNA mutation or chromosome anomaly. The genetic change is confined solely to the germ line (the cells which produce the gametes) of the parent, so that the other cells in the person's body have the normal genetic complement. This means that clinically normal people with normal gene test results can still have undetected abnormal genes in their gonads and pass these on to their children. For example, in Duchenne muscular dystrophy, a female who does not show the same mutation as her affected son on a blood test may still have a 20 % risk of being a gonadal mosaic and having another affected son. Another example would be where clinically normal parents have more than one child with an autosomal dominant condition such as achondroplasia. Currently, there is no way of testing to see if someone is a gonadal mosaic. Because of this phenomenon, some clinically normal parents who do not appear to be affected or carriers may seek PND or PGD.

Key Points
- Couples who wish to consider PGD must be seen by a clinical geneticist first to confirm the genetic diagnosis, understand the mode of inheritance of the particular disorder, calculate the recurrence risk within a family, establish whether there is any risk to other relatives and to review all reproductive options including PGD.
- Most numerical chromosome abnormalities are sporadic and usually result in miscarriage.
- Balanced reciprocal and Robertsonian translocations are the most common chromosomal rearrangements.
- For PGD to be possible for a single-gene disorder, the gene mutation must have been identified and be known to be disease-causing rather than variant of uncertain significance. Linkage studies may also be helpful.
- With metabolic disorders, PGD is different from prenatal diagnosis where testing can be done on enzyme assay alone. For some rare metabolic disorders, identifying gene mutations may be very problematic. If linkage studies cannot be performed, couples may find it hard to understand why they can have prenatal diagnosis but not PGD.

Further Reading

Bradley-Smith G, Hope S, Firth H, Hurst J. Oxford handbook of genetics. Oxford/New York: OUP; 2010.

Firth H, Hurst J. Oxford desk reference: clinical genetics. Oxford/New York: OUP; 2005.

Harper P. Practical genetic counselling. 7th ed. London: Hodder Arnold; 2010.

National genetics education and development centre. http://www.geneticseducation.nhs.uk/.

Read A, Donnai D. New clinical genetics. Bloxham/Oxfordshire: Scion; 2007.

Turnpenny P, Ellard S. Emery's elements of medical genetics. 12th ed. Edinburgh/London/New York: Elsevier; 2005.

Chapter 3
Genetic Counselling and Its Role in PGD

Alison Lashwood

PGD has now been available for over two decades and the number of patients treated has increased annually. The process is by nature complex and requires a high level of clinical and laboratory understanding, including the practicalities of assisted reproduction treatment, some aspects of which may be unfamiliar to even experienced geneticists and genetic counsellors. The PGD Consortium of the European Society of Human Reproduction and Embryology (ESHRE) and the Preimplantation Genetic Diagnosis International Society (PGDIS) recommend that acceptable practice requires that the counselling should be offered to all couples requesting PGD and is provided in a nondirective manner by an appropriately qualified professional. The combined skills of genetic counsellors and clinical geneticists from accredited genetic centres, working together with specialists in assisted reproductive medicine, should ensure that patients receive a high-quality service in PGD.

Most couples will have experienced the loss of a child or a pregnancy and possibly had prenatal diagnosis (PND). They are generally united in their wish to have a child that is

A. Lashwood, MSc, RGN, RSCN, DIPHV
Clinical Genetics Department, Guy's and St. Thomas' Hospital
NHS Foundation Trust, 7th Floor, Borough Wing, Guy's Hospital,
Great Maze Pond, London SE1 9RT, UK
e-mail: alison.lashwood@gstt.nhs.uk

T. El-Toukhy, P. Braude (eds.), *Preimplantation Genetic Diagnosis in Clinical Practice*, DOI 10.1007/978-1-4471-2948-6_3, © Springer-Verlag London 2014

biologically related, but is unaffected by the genetic disorder within the family. The most commonly cited reason for using PGD is to avoid termination of pregnancy. For others, the advantage of PGD is the knowledge that from very early on in gestation, the pregnancy is unaffected. Therefore, it is an essential part of the PGD genetic counselling process to establish the reason for choosing PGD to ensure that couples' expectations can reasonably be met.

The aim of genetic counselling is to deliver accurate information alongside the support given to patients to enable them to make the most appropriate decision for them personally, whilst ensuring as far as possible that no pressure is applied from clinical professionals involved in their care. Genetic counselling services vary in structure being delivered by a combination of medically qualified clinical geneticists and genetic counsellors with a nursing or science background and a Master's level degree in a related field.

Genetic Counselling Before a Treatment Cycle

Before a couple is referred for PGD, they will have usually consulted a clinical geneticist to discuss the implications of the genetic condition affecting their family. Such consultations provide patients with information about the condition, recurrence risks, contemporary appropriate genetic testing, discussion of reproductive options, organisation of family follow-up and support in coming to terms with the diagnosis.

Prior to the start of a PGD treatment cycle, it is important that couples:

- Discuss their family history and reason for requesting PGD
- Understand their genetic risk
- Know what alternative reproductive options are available
- Understand the PGD process and the side effects of treatment

- Understand the limitations of testing and success rates
- Consider the physical, psychological and financial impact of treatment
- Receive a written summary of the consultation and relevant patient information leaflets

Genetic Counselling Is Not the Same as Infertility Counselling

Although IVF is used in both procedures, and some couples may have experienced childlessness due to repeated miscarriage, or incidentally as result of their genetic condition, e.g. Klinefelter syndrome or Turner syndrome, the expertise of the genetic counsellor is in helping couples to better understand their genetic condition and prepare for PGD as a means of avoiding transmission.

Counselling Issues Specific to PGD

Welfare of the Child

In accordance with the UK Human Fertilisation and Embryology Act (2008), centres treating couples are responsible for ensuring any assisted reproductive treatment offered and must take account of the welfare of any children born as a result. Some couples requesting PGD will be affected with the genetic disorder in their family and have associated clinical symptoms. A condition such as cystic fibrosis may be life limiting or, in the case of Huntington disease (HD), associated with long-term progressive disability. Such issues require discussion with the couple to establish how they would manage in the event that one parent is no longer able to care for a child and the unaffected partner becomes the carer or the affected parent dies whilst the child is at a young age.

Impact of Treatment on the Family

A family caring for a child with a disability needs to consider the impact of travel to appointments and the rigorous demands of the treatment schedule. The risk of ovarian hyperstimulation syndrome with the possibility of hospitalisation must also be considered. Couples should always be encouraged to establish support networks to ensure backup if there are complications associated with treatment.

Choices at Embryo Transfer

Number of Embryos to Be Transferred

The number of embryos used in transfer continues to court controversy in the world of assisted reproduction because of the perceived improvement in chances of cycle success with the transfer of two embryos versus the increased chance of multiple birth. Twins and triplets add another dimension of difficulty to couples seeking PGD; as well as the physical hazard to both mother and babies associated with twin or triplet birth; the social and psychological impact of a multiple birth is considerable. Many of the couples that request PGD already may be caring for children with disabilities. The introduction of more than one further child therefore needs careful consideration in relation to the potential impact on the family. Prolonged hospital stay and the risk of damage or disability from prematurity may further add to the burden.

Carrier Status

Since embryos that carry one copy of a recessive gene or females in X-linked disorders generally are unaffected by the disorder being tested, they can be recommended for transfer. Excluding carrier embryos reduces the cohort of transferable embryos which in turn could compromise the success rate of treatment. Couples are usually fully informed of the disease status of all their embryos and should also have been made aware whether there is any significant risk to transfer of carriers – see below. However, this information may conflict with recommendations for carrier testing in childhood, an issue that has been debated within the genetics community for many years. The report "Genetic Testing in Childhood" recommends that unless there are clinical benefits to testing minors, testing for carrier status should be delayed until a child is old enough to understand the implications and be part of the decision making. In addition, since prenatal diagnosis generally is offered as a means of confirming the PGD result, or should that be declined, by umbilical cord blood testing at birth, it is important that the issue of childhood testing is discussed with couples before carrier status is attributed to an embryo, fetus or neonate.

Sex Selection

Sex selection on social grounds is prohibited in most European countries and in the UK under the terms of the HFE Act (2008), but is freely allowed in some countries (Jordan) or condoned in others (USA). However, when undertaking PGD for X-linked disorders, the laboratory will be able to determine the sex of the embryos as well as their disease status. In some conditions where carrier females may have a clinical phenotype (e.g. as in the case of Fragile X or haemophilia A/B), there may be good clinical grounds for not transferring carrier embryos. Embryos that are genetically suitable for transfer should always be prioritised on the basis of their morphological quality and potential for implantation. However, in the absence of a clinical phenotype associated with carrier status, couples could be aware of the sex of their embryos and should be given the option *NOT* to know the sex of their embryos.

Genetic Counselling After a PGD Cycle

Successful Cycle and Confirmation of Diagnosis

Following a successful PGD cycle and confirmatory first trimester viability scans (Chap. 9), the couple should be contacted by the genetic counsellor to discuss the option of confirmatory prenatal diagnosis. All PGD cases have a small risk of misdiagnosis, which will vary depending upon the test used, the skill of the centre offering treatment and the condition for which PGD was offered. Chorionic villus sampling (CVS), amniocentesis and anomaly scanning are all possible and widely available options. For many couples confirmatory testing is difficult issue to confront, as they are reluctant to put the pregnancy at risk from invasive testing. As many couples have used PGD to avoid the issue of termination, the prospect of having to face this possibility after prenatal diagnosis leads many to decline confirmatory testing. Collecting an umbilical cord blood sample at birth provides an alternative means to confirm successful avoidance of the genetic condition, although many centres will not offer this option in PGD for Huntington disease. As these couples often decline prenatal diagnosis, confirmatory testing at birth could result in mutation detection in a child, should a misdiagnosis have occurred and would contravene current clinical guidelines which advocate against testing of minors for late onset conditions since the child has not had an opportunity to consent to such testing.

Unsuccessful Cycle and Follow-Up

Around 30 % of PGD cycles will not result in embryo transfer due to:

- Poor response to ovarian stimulation
- Failure of fertilisation
- Poor embryo quality incompatible with biopsy
- Absence of genetically suitable embryos for transfer

Other couples will have a negative pregnancy test after embryo transfer or suffer an early pregnancy loss following a positive test. Each of these is a disappointing and often distressing outcome for couples. These couples should always be offered a follow-up appointment as soon as possible to discuss the outcome of the cycle, and where appropriate to discuss any future treatment planned. Some may have embryos cryopreserved for additional attempts at transfer, whilst for others the advice may be that further cycles are not recommended where the chance of success is considered too low. Such discussions need sensitive counselling and involvement of the rest of the PGD team. Genetic counsellors can support the couples at or after these consultations and liaise with the couple's local genetic centre where necessary.

Paediatric Follow-Up

In most cases, a successful PGD cycle will result in an ongoing pregnancy and a healthy live born infant. Although PGD is a well-established clinical service, outcome data on babies born is limited (see Chap. 11 and 18). Long-term follow-up and data collection have been recommended since the early days of PGD. The ESHRE PGD consortium recommends paediatric review at birth, 1 and 2 years of age. This can be organised via the PGD centre involved in the treatment of a couple or on a more local basis following referral to a paediatrician.

Recent ESHRE PGD consortium data reported that no malformations were detected in 95 % of PGD babies. Abnormalities were varied and ranged from significant cardiac abnormalities to mild syndactyly. Longer-term studies seem to reflect that growth and developmental parameters in PGD children are equivalent to IVF/ICSI children and normal controls.

Key Points
- Genetic counselling is an integral part of the PGD process.
- Genetic counselling is not the same as fertility counselling.
- Couples should have access to genetics expertise from the point of referral to monitoring of babies born following treatment.
- In accordance with recommended practice guidelines, appropriately qualified personnel should be employed to work as members of the PGD team.

Further Reading

Ad Hoc Committee on Genetic Counseling American Society for Human Genetics. Genetic counselling. Am J Hum Genet. 1975;27:240–2.

Banerjee I, Shevlin M, Taranissi M, Thornhill A, Abdalla H, Ozturk O, et al. Health of children conceived after preimplantation genetic diagnosis: a preliminary outcome study. Reprod Biomed Online. 2008;16:376–81.

British Medical Association. Human genetics: choice and responsibility. Oxford: Oxford University Press; 1998.

Desmyttere S, De Schepper J, Nekkebroeck J, De Vos A, De Rycke M, Staessen C, et al. Two-year auxological and medical outcome of singletons born after embryo biopsy applied in preimplantation genetic diagnosis or preimplantation genetic screening. Hum Reprod. 2009;24:470–6.

ESHRE. PGD consortium publications I-X. Accessed at: http://www.eshre.eu/ESHRE/English/Specialty-Groups/Data-collection-Consortia/PGD-Consortium/PGD-Consortium-Publications/page.aspx/217. Accessed on 28 Aug 2013.

Kessler S. Psychological aspects of genetic counselling. XI. Nondirectiveness revisited. Am J Med Genet. 1997;72(2):164–71.

Lashwood A, Kanabar D, El-Toukhy T, Kavalier F. Paediatric outcome from birth onwards after preimplantation genetic diagnosis. J Med Genet. 2007;44 Suppl 1:S28.

Nekkebroeck J, Bonduelle M, Desmyttere S, Van den Broeck W, Ponjaert-Kristoffersen I. Mental and psychomotor development of 2-year-old children born after preimplantation genetic diagnosis/screening. Hum Reprod. 2008;23:1560–6.

Nekkebroeck J, Bonduelle M, Desmyttere S, Van den Broeck W, Ponjaert-Kristoffersen I. Socioemotional and language development of 2-year-old children born after PGD/PGS, and parental well-being. Hum Reprod. 2008;23:1849–57.

Palomba ML, Monni G, Lai R, Cau G, Olla G, Cao A. Psychological implications and acceptability of preimplantation diagnosis. Hum Reprod. 1994;9:360–2.

Preimplantation Genetic Diagnosis International Society (PGDIS). Guidelines for good practice in PGD: programme requirements and laboratory quality assurance. RBM Online. 2008;16:134–47.

Thornhill AR, deDie-Smulders CE, Geraedts JP, Harper JC, Harton GL, Lavery SA, Moutou C, Robinson MD, Schmutzler AG, Scriven PS, Sermon KD, Wilton L. ESHRE PGD consortium "best practice guidelines for clinical preimplantation genetic diagnosis (PGD) and preimplantation genetic screening (PGS)". Hum Reprod. 2005; 20:35–48.

Chapter 4
Complex Issues in PGD

Alison Lashwood and Genevieve Say

The process of PGD is complex and can be challenging for both professionals and patients alike. However, there are additional complexities that arise and may not be obvious to the practitioner new to PGD. Each centre offering PGD will work within its own practical, ethical and moral framework and, where present, in accordance with specific national regulations. This chapter will address some of the issues that require further consideration when providing a PGD clinical service.

Late-Onset Conditions

Preimplantation genetic diagnosis for conditions with an adult onset presents the PGD team with a unique set of issues that require special consideration. Predictive testing is

A. Lashwood, MSc, RGN, RSCN, DIPHV (✉)
Clinical Genetics Department, Guy's and St. Thomas Hospital NHS
Foundation Trust, 7th Floor Borough Wing, Guy's Hospital,
Great Maze Pond, London SE1 9RT, UK
e-mail: alison.lashwood@gstt.nhs.uk

G. Say, BA (Psychol), GradDipGC
Clinical Genetics Department, Guy's and St. Thomas NHS Trust,
Level 7 Borough Wing, Guy's Hospital, Great Maze Pond,
London SE1 9RT, UK
e-mail: genevieve.say@gstt.nhs.uk

T. El-Toukhy, P. Braude (eds.), *Preimplantation Genetic Diagnosis in Clinical Practice*, DOI 10.1007/978-1-4471-2948-6_4,
© Springer-Verlag London 2014

available for a number of adult-onset disorders such as Huntington disease, (HD) which forms a good example of this group and its problems. PGD is available not only for those who know that they have inherited the HD gene mutation (direct testing) but also for those who are at 50 % risk of inheriting the disease (exclusion testing).

Although symptom onset is usually well into adulthood, the clinical, psychological and practical implications of such conditions are so profound that PGD for HD is one of the leading treatment requests. Uptake of prenatal diagnosis for HD is low perhaps because as a late onset condition, the decision about termination of pregnancy is even more difficult for many couples, and there continues to be the hope of a cure in time for the next generation.

HD Direct Testing PGD

PGD by direct testing has been available since 1998 and should only be undertaken when a positive presymptomatic test result is available. Individuals who have requested a presymptomatic genetic test will have done so for varied reasons: the 'need to know', making decisions about starting a family, lifestyle choices, planning for the future, 'for the sake of children' and for some because they may have had concerns that they are showing symptoms. As professionals were concerned about the impact of such testing, international guidelines were drawn up to help prepare a person at risk for the result. Those who opt not to undergo testing often state that the overriding reason behind nonparticipation is concern about their ability to cope with a bad news result. Undertaking direct testing an embryos in the absence of a presymptomatic test presents difficult ethical and medical dilemmas which can be avoided by indirect (exclusion) testing.

HD Exclusion PGD

Exclusion testing PGD has been licensed in the UK by the HFEA since 2002. The aim here is to exclude embryos that carry the high-risk (50 %) grandparental allele. Those requesting exclusion testing are at 50 % risk of inheriting the gene and have chosen not to have a presymptomatic test usually out of concern for their ability to cope with the practical issues associated with an adverse result. It is possible to develop a test that excludes the high-risk grandparental copy of chromosome 4 which contains the HD allele, without disclosing the HD status of the at risk partner.

A number of arguments against such testing have been raised including concern over the invasive nature of PGD to a woman who may not require treatment if there is no risk of passing on the gene, the destruction of embryos that may not have a genetic risk, and whether it is the best use of health resources when a couple does not have a proven genetic risk.

Confirmation of PGD Results in Late-Onset Disorders

Couples who successfully conceive an ongoing pregnancy after PGD for single-gene disorders with childhood onset or for chromosomal rearrangements usually are offered confirmatory prenatal testing due to the associated misdiagnosis risk. As the misdiagnosis risk is low, most couples opt not to undergo prenatal diagnosis and continue with the pregnancy untested. Analysis of cord blood at birth is an alternative method of PGD confirmation.

Confirmation of diagnosis for autosomal dominant late-onset disorders raises the particular issue of presymptomatic testing in a child, since the diagnosis of the presence or absence of the gene either at prenatal testing or in cord blood changes the right of the child to an 'open future' and thus conflicts with recommended childhood testing guidelines.

Cancer Susceptibility

Genetic testing for cancer susceptibility genes is now more widely available, and many who opt for testing are of reproductive age. In response to demand, a number of genetic cancer predisposition syndromes have now been licensed by the Human Fertilisation and Embryology Authority (HFEA) for PGD, which include:

- BRCA1 and BRCA2 (breast and ovarian cancer)
- Lynch syndrome (bowel, endometrial and ovarian cancer)
- Familial Adenomatous Polyposis (FAP) (thousands of bowel polyps with malignant potential)
- Li-Fraumeni syndrome (breast cancer and other soft-tissue tumours)
- Neurofibromatosis type 2 (schwannomas)

Such pathogenic mutations in monogenic disorders are said to be not fully penetrant; not all who carry the pathogenic mutation will develop the disease. For example, BRCA carrier status confers a lifetime risk of up to 80 % for breast cancer and up to 50 % for ovarian cancer. Cancer predisposition syndromes are often adult onset, most are not fully penetrant, and all have some degree of risk-reducing management available. However, compared to sporadic cancers, hereditary cancers often manifest at a younger age and imply an increased risk of developing multiple primary tumours.

Besides penetrance, the fact that risk-reducing strategies are available for those who carry mutations divides opinion as to the appropriateness of PGD as a reproductive option.

However, risk-reducing management includes various types of invasive screening and prophylactic surgery, such as mastectomy, oophorectomy or colectomy, which may impact psychological wellbeing and quality of life.

Prenatal testing (PND) for cancer predisposition syndromes is rarely requested. Whilst many of those at risk feel pregnancy termination for BRCA is justified, some health professionals are reluctant to offer prenatal testing for some cancer predisposition syndromes due to the lack of penetrance. PGD is an appealing alternative for those couples who see embryo selection as more acceptable than pregnancy termination. As the cancer predisposition syndromes manifest with such variability, acceptability levels of PGD are also variable among those at risk. Acceptability is largely determined by a couple's perception of severity of cancer. However, as cancer is common, individuals born following PGD treatment, whilst not at high risk for the specific cancers tested for, would still have the 1 in 3 population risk of developing some type of cancer over their lifetime. A review of literature shows that awareness of PGD is low among those with cancer predisposition syndromes.

Infertility and PGD

Over 30 % of patients referred for PGD will also have an underlying fertility problem. The cause of subfertility may be linked to the genetic condition, e.g. congenital absence of the vas deferens (CBAVD) or chromosome rearrangements. Whilst the use of PGD as an adjunct to Assisted Reproductive Technology (ART) may be clinically justified, careful consideration of the benefits and costs is required.

According to the ESHRE consortium, around 15 % of embryos following PGD will be excluded due to technical failure to make a diagnosis (non-diagnosis risk) and as such PGD will reduce the number of embryos available for transfer above the number diagnosed as affected. This issue may be less relevant when embryo numbers are abundant, but in cycles with few embryos, testing may compromise the chance of embryo transfer and hence chances of pregnancy. Detailed discussion about the impact of the transfer of an affected embryo following an IVF cycle needs to be weighed against the reduced success rate of adding PGD. For example, in the case of a couple carrying a balanced chromosome translocation where the most likely outcome of an unbalanced conception is miscarriage, the couple may prefer to try IVF alone and maximise the number of embryos available for transfer or cryopreservation and consider prenatal diagnosis as an alternative if concerned about continuing genetic abnormality. In addition preparation and workup for PGD takes additional time, so those concerned about timeframes, which is a common concern in the pursuit of fertility treatment, IVF without PGD may be a preferable option. However, some centres offering fertility treatment are uncomfortable offering ART to couples with a high genetic risk.

It is not uncommon for there to be so few embryos available that proceeding with genetic testing may simply remove any likelihood of transfer. Taking into account the risk of non-diagnosis, it may be preferable to go ahead with transfer anyway, especially if the couple is prepared to consider Prenatal Diagnosis (PND) in these circumstances.

Where PGD has gone ahead and reveals there are only affected embryos available, there is the potential for a request to transfer anyway especially if this is the couple's only chance of having a baby. These scenarios are not that infrequent and merit discussion with the couple ahead of treatment.

Gamete Donation and PGD

In the context of genetics the use of donated gametes serves two purposes; to enable people who have a genetic disorder to avoid passing on the gene to their children, or to enable those who have a genetic disorder causing infertility, to become parents.

Donated gametes for infertility are generally used when the female partner has low ovarian reserve or premature ovarian failure, or the male partner is azoospermic. In PGD it may be the fertile partner who carries the genetic risk and additional effort is required in donor matching, making the already difficult process of procuring a suitable donated egg or sperm additionally complex.

Donors may be sought through recruitment of anonymous altruistic donors or by payment for gametes from national or international donor banks if regulations so allow. Besides the standard screening tests to eliminate common conditions such as cystic fibrosis, thalassaemia, Tay-Sachs and sickle-cell disease, depending on the population risks, an additional blood sample will be required from the donor for the development or validation of the specific PGD tests to be used. If anonymous donors are used, special arrangements have to be made to access the sample through the centre that provided the donor. Access to such samples is not always possible and may result in PGD being unavailable to the couple. The donor must also be informed that their gametes are being used for PGD, and specific permission for the blood test and the embryo test is generally required. Couples recruiting donors through family members need to ensure the donor does not carry the same familial condition that is being tested by PGD.

PGD for Social Reasons

Sex Selection

In many countries use of PGD is regulated by law, and in most, as in the UK, its use to sex embryos for non-medical reasons is illegal. However, couples going through PGD for a serious genetic condition will sometimes express a preference that a certain gender embryo is replaced if both male and female unaffected embryos are available. Requests for a certain gender of embryo may be linked to the condition itself, such as in haemophilia where a carrier female may manifest the disorder and the severity may be difficult to predict. However, requests may come from couples with an affected son such that only female embryos are transferred. In the case of X-linked Duchenne muscular dystrophy, for example, a couple may not want their affected son to see a healthy younger brother develop the ability to reach the physical potential that the affected sibling is unable to do. They may believe that a daughter is less likely to be compared in physical pursuits. Each of these needs to be considered on its merits, for medical, social, psychological and legal factors.

Genetic Risk for Future Generations

Most female carriers of X-linked conditions and carriers of autosomal recessive disorders or chromosome rearrangements will have no associated health problems. The aim of PGD is help couples conceive a *healthy* child. However, couples often request exclusion of carrier embryos to avoid the risk of having affected grandchildren. This is an understandable concern and perhaps reflects the feelings of significant levels of guilt and sense of responsibility to their future children. On the other hand, those who have reservations about PGD being the pursuit of 'designer babies' may cite this approach as eugenic.

After discussion about the limited success rates of PGD, most couples are happy to have a carrier embryo transferred if it represents the best chance of having a healthy child. They often have faith also that technology and options will improve significantly by the time their children are confronted with reproductive risks.

Key Points
- Complex issues arise as part of the PGD process.
- Patients' requests for PGD may not solely be made on the basis of the genetic disorder.
- PGD must be practised in accordance within the regulatory framework of a specific country and recommended practice guidelines.

Further Reading

Braude P. Preimplantation diagnosis for genetic susceptibility. N Engl J Med. 2006;355(6):541.

Braude P, De Wert G, Evers-Kiebooms G, Pettigrew R, Geraedts JP. Non-disclosure preimplantation genetic diagnosis for Huntington's disease: practical and ethical dilemmas. Prenat Diagn. 1998;18(13): 1422–6.

British Society of Human Genetics. Report on the genetic testing of children. 2010. http://www.bshg.org.uk/GTOC_Booklet_Final_new.pdf.

Ford D, Easton DF, Stratton M, Narod S, Goldgar D, Devilee P, Bishop DT, Weber B, Lenoir G, Chang-Claude J, Sobol H, Teare MD, Struewing J, Arason A, Scherneck S, Peto J, Rebbeck TR, Tonin P, Neuhausen S, Barkardottir R, Eyfjord J, Lynch H, Ponder BA, Gayther SA, Zelada-Hedman M, et al. Genetic heterogeneity and penetrance analysis of the BRCA1 and BRCA2 genes in breast cancer families. The Breast Cancer Linkage Consortium. Am J Hum Genet. 1998;62(3):676–89.

HFEA Consultation Document. Choices and boundaries. Should people be able to select embryos free from an inherited susceptibility to cancer? 2005. http://www.hfea.gov.uk/docs/Choices_and_Boundaries.pdf.

Hurley K, Rubin L, Werner-Lin A, Sagi M, Kemel Y, Stern R, et al. Incorporating information regarding preimplantation genetic diagnosis into discussions concerning testing and risk management for BRCA1/2 mutations. Cancer. 2012;118(24):6270–7.

Lashwood A, Flinter F. Clinical and counselling implications of preimplantation genetic diagnosis for Huntington's disease in the UK. Hum Fertil. 2001;4(4):235–8.

Macleod R, Tibben A, Frontali M, Evers-Kiebooms G, Jones A, Martinez-Descales A, Roos R. Editorial Committee and Working Group 'Genetic Testing and Counselling' of the European Huntington Disease Network. Recommendations for the predictive genetic test in Huntington's disease. Clin Genet. 2012. doi:10.1111/j.1399-0004.2012.01900.x.

Ormondroyd E, Donnelly L, Moynihan C, Savona C, Bancroft E, Evans G, et al. Attitudes to reproductive genetic testing in women who had a positive BRCA test before having children: a qualitative analysis. Eur J Human Genet. 2012;20:4–10.

Quinn G, Pal T, Murphy D, Vadaparampil S, Kumar A. High-risk consumers' perceptions of preimplantation genetic diagnosis for hereditary cancers: a systematic review and meta-analysis. Genet Med. 2012;14(2):191–200.

HFEA Consultation Document. Sex Selection: Choice and Responsibility In Human Reproduction. 2003. http://www.hfea.gov.uk/docs/Sex_Selection_choice_and_responsibility.pdf.

Thies U, Zuhlke C, Bockel B, Schroder K. Prenatal diagnosis of Huntington's disease (HD): experiences with six cases and PCR. Prenat Diagn. 1992;12:1055–61.

Chapter 5
Assisted Reproductive Care for PGD Patients

Willem M.J.A. Verpoest and Christine E.M. de Die-Smulders

Assisted reproductive care for patients requesting PGD is for many reasons beyond that provided to patients undergoing reproductive treatment for non-genetic indications. A major difference is the fact that up to 70 % of PGD patients are not documented to have a fertility problem. Another consideration is that, although the ideal outcome is a healthy singleton live born, there is a shift in focus to an optimum number of good quality oocytes, embryos or blastocysts for biopsy.

Willem M.J.A. Verpoest, MD, PhD (✉)
Department of Reproductive Medicine and Gynaecology,
Universitair Ziekenhuis Brussel of the Vrije Universiteit Brussel,
Centre for Reproductive Medicine, 101 Laarbeeklaan,
Brussels B-1090, Belgium
e-mail: willem.verpoest@uzbrussel.be

C.E.M. de Die-Smulders, MD, PhD
Department of Clinical Genetics, University Hospital Maastricht,
5800, Maastricht 6202 AZ, The Netherlands
e-mail: c.dedie@mumc.nl

T. El-Toukhy, P. Braude (eds.), *Preimplantation Genetic Diagnosis in Clinical Practice*, DOI 10.1007/978-1-4471-2948-6_5, © Springer-Verlag London 2014

Basic Assisted Reproductive Techniques Involved in PGD

Patient Management

Specific requirements are essential for both the clinical and laboratory setting of PGD (see Chap. 6). A multidisciplinary setting involving clinical geneticists and reproductive specialists, and when necessary, physicians, neurologists, paediatricians, oncologists, obstetricians and internal medicine or other specialists, is required to cover the range of medical issues involved in the management of PGD patients. The patient and/or his/her relatives often suffer with genetic disorders that may require special attention with regard to periconceptional care and risks that need to be addressed prior to start of PGD treatment. Psychological counselling is required in many cases including when PGD for HLA compatibility testing is being considered.

The pretreatment workup needs to be completed as for patients undergoing routine IVF treatment without PGD. This includes ovarian reserve testing in order to determine the optimum stimulation protocol and serological testing for infectious diseases as required by local legislation. Sperm analysis for the male is essential, most specifically for men carrying a hereditary condition potentially associated with reduced spermatogenesis such as myotonic dystrophy type 1 and balanced structural or numerical chromosomal aberrations, including Klinefelter syndrome.

Consent by the patient and her partner with regard to embryo selection by PGD is important. The informed consent form should include procedure-specific information, risk of false negative diagnosis, advice on prenatal testing following PGD as well as issues regarding the fate of embryos that are judged not genetically transferable. Specific consent is required when an exceptional transfer decision is made, e.g. when diagnosis is inconclusive or failed, or the genetic diagnosis deviates from the one agreed on originally to be allowed for transfer.

Female Fertility Issues

Ovarian Reserve

Women with X chromosome aberrations are at risk of reduced ovarian reserve. Assessment of ovarian reserve is essential whenever numerical or structural chromosomal abnormalities aberrations are involved especially those involving the X chromosome.

The most sensitive test currently available is serum anti-Müllerian hormone (AMH) analysis. AMH is produced by the granulosa cells surrounding the oocytes and is quantitatively related to the number of oocytes available. Alternative testing includes early follicular phase serum follicle-stimulating hormone (FSH) analysis or the antral follicle count on ultrasound.

Women who are expected to have poor ovarian response at ovarian stimulation, or have proven to have done so in the past, should be counselled about the reduced chances of success, as the number of oocytes collected is significantly associated with reproductive outcome in PGD (Chap. 12). There is no fixed threshold for the number of oocytes required; moderate ovarian response is associated with good reproductive outcome, especially in younger patients.

Body Mass Index

Obesity

Obesity leads to anovulation and is commonly associated with polycystic ovarian syndrome (PCOS). Obesity and PCOS share several pathophysiological characteristics including insulin resistance and hyperandrogenemia. A distinction between gynecoid obesity (esthetic) and android obesity (metabolic) is important at first consultation. In addition, there are ethnic variations in obesity. White Caucasians are considered obese above a body mass index (BMI) of 30, whereas Asians are considered obese above a BMI of 25.

TABLE 5.1 Non-genetic factors affecting ovarian response and embryo implantation

Conditions that could potentially affect ovarian response are:
Endometriosis
Ovarian cysts
Use of certain medication
Obesity/anorexia
Polycystic ovarian syndrome
Conditions that potentially affect embryo implantation are:
Intrauterine abnormalities including polyps, fibroids, adenomyosis and Müllerian duct abnormalities
Endometritis
Thrombophilia
Antiphospholipid syndrome
Thyroid function abnormalities
Psychological stress

Underweight

The onset and regularity of menstrual function necessitates maintaining the body weight above a critical level, and therefore a critical amount of body fat is important. Acute weight loss and anorexia nervosa can lead to a hypogonadotrophic anovulatory state and can have an effect on oocyte number and quality in assisted reproductive treatment. Thin patients have a propensity to hyperstimulate easily.

Female Infertility Not Related to the Genetic Condition

Up to 70 % of couples presenting at a PGD clinic have no documented infertility. However, gynaecological pathology can be present or become obvious during the course of pretreatment workup or the treatment itself. Such pathology (Table 5.1) needs to be addressed in a similar fashion as in patients having routine IVF treatment, in order to optimise ovarian response, oocyte quality as well as embryo implantation and pregnancy.

Female Infertility Related to Specific Genetic Conditions

A number of genetic conditions may cause a depletion of ovarian reserve. This needs to be taken into account when preparing for PGD treatment.

Fragile X Mental Retardation Protein 1 (FMR1) Premutation (Fragile X Syndrome)

This condition is caused by a dynamic CGG repeat expansion in the 5′ untranslated region of the FMRP gene. A premutation is defined as more than 55 but less than 200 CGG repeats. The natural history of altered ovarian function associated with fragile X syndrome premutation is not entirely known, but it is assumed that it induces accelerated follicular atresia. As a result, the average age at menopause is significantly lower, and there is a higher incidence of premature ovarian failure (POF) in fragile X syndrome premutation carriers compared to noncarriers. There appears to be a significant influence of repeat size on the risk for ovarian failure, with increasing prevalence of POF and decreasing age at menopause correlating with increasing repeat size. However, this relationship seems to be non-linear as the risk of POF appears to plateau or even decrease in carriers of over 100 repeats. The ideal stimulation protocol in these patients is not evident; different strategies may need to be explored, and often poor response cannot be avoided.

Myotonic Dystrophy Type I (DM1; Steinert Syndrome)

Ovarian function in affected women has generally been considered normal, but poor ovarian reserve, oligomenorrhoea, abortions and early menopause have been reported in several studies. Nevertheless, larger studies looking into reproductive function of DM1 patients after PGD are still required.

Chromosomal Abnormalities

Miscarriage is increased in couples where one of the partners is carrying a balanced reciprocal or Robertsonian chromosomal translocation. It is unclear whether female carriers of balanced autosomal translocations carry an increased risk of reduced ovarian response and specific autosomal translocations associated with POF have not been established. On the other hand, defective follicular production or excessive apoptosis has been reported in patients with a balanced translocation involving the long arm of the X chromosome. Women lacking an X chromosome (Turner syndrome) are known to be infertile with streak ovaries and are not normally offered PGD. Occasionally, women carrying an extra X chromosome could be at risk of reduced ovarian reserve and POF.

BRCA Mutation Carriers

Ovarian stimulation for reproductive treatment or fertility preservation exposes the female to increased levels of estrogens, hence theoretically could increase the risk of developing or recurrence of certain hereditary gynaecological cancers such as breast and ovarian cancer in BRCA1 or 2 mutation carriers and TP53 mutation carriers and other hereditary oncological disorders. However, such an increased risk is yet to be demonstrated in large studies. Furthermore, and rather paradoxically, female BRCA1 carriers are thought to have a reduced ovarian response, despite the absence of clinically obvious fertility problems.

Low-dose ovarian stimulation has thus far only been studied in patients actually affected by cancer and requesting fertility preservation. In view of the increasing demand for PGD and/or fertility preservation in this patient group, studies are needed to improve reproductive results and coordinate registration, counselling and follow-up of these patients.

Male Fertility Issues

Sperm analysis is required for all males entering the PGD programme. In men with very poor sperm quality, cryopreservation of sperm is justified as backup for use in PGD treatment and as a fertility preservation measure.

Klinefelter Syndrome

A number of genetic conditions are associated with reduced sperm quality. Klinefelter syndrome is associated with testicular atrophy and is the most common genetic cause of non-obstructive azoospermia. Spermatogenesis may be preserved to some extent in these patients. Thus, spermatozoa could be obtained in many Klinefelter patients undergoing ICSI and testicular sperm extraction (TESE). Although testicular volume and serum follicle-stimulating hormone (FSH) level are not reliable predictors of spermatogenesis, clinical examination by orchidometry remains important in these patients in order to determine feasibility of testicular biopsy.

Chromosome Rearrangements

Assessment of sperm quality is essential whenever structural chromosomal anomalies, such as translocations, are involved, as it is known that they are more often associated with oligoasthenozoospermia or sometimes even azoospermia. The recurrent Robertsonian translocation between chromosomes 13 and 14 is well known to be associated with male infertility and a relatively frequent indication for PGD.

Congenital Absence of the Vas Deferens (CBAVD)

CBAVD is a type of obstructive azoospermia in which both vasa deferentia are absent, and the seminal vesicles are atrophic or absent as are large portions of the epididymis. This condition is most commonly diagnosed in presence of azoospermia in otherwise normal men, either on clinical examination or by scrotal ultrasound. In men affected with cystic fibrosis, 97–98 % are found to have CBAVD. Conversely, in men who have been diagnosed with CBAVD and who are not affected with cystic fibrosis (CF), a mutation of the CFTR gene is frequent. In those cases where no mutation is identified, there remains a suspicion of the presence of an as yet unknown mutation or combination of alleles. Many CBAVD patients do not have significant lung or pancreatic disease as the homozygous mutation(s) they carry is thought either to be associated with milder disease or to have a different tissue-specific effect. Spermatogenesis is normal in most males with CBAVD, although occasionally a mutation in the CFTR gene can be associated with defective spermatogenesis. Extended CF testing should be conducted because of the added risk of an occult CF mutation which could have potentially serious consequences in the offspring with a known CF carrier female.

Myotonic Dystrophy

Although secondary sexual development is usually normal, males affected by myotonic dystrophy type 1 have an increased risk of hypogonadism, raised FSH levels and lower testosterone levels. As a result, sperm quality is on average worse than in non-affected men, probably due to progressive seminiferous tubular destruction. The CTG expansion associated with DM1 causes transcriptional silencing of the flanking *Six5* gene. A decrease in *Six5* gene expression has been associated with deficient spermatogenesis and a progressive decrease in testicular mass with age.

Medical Conditions Related to Carrier State of the Genetic Condition

Genetic disorders may interfere with and complicate PGD treatment. This is especially true for couples affected with an autosomal dominant disorder or female carriers of an

X-linked disorder. Genetic disorders may also give rise to increased risks in pregnancy or concerns regarding the prognosis of the diseased parent at the long term. It is of paramount importance to identify the high-risk patients prior to starting PGD treatment.

Effects of the Genetic Disorder on PGD Treatment and Subsequent Pregnancy

Disorders Affecting the Cardiovascular System

In women with disorders affecting the cardiovascular system, such as Marfan syndrome or Ehlers-Danlos syndrome type IV (the vascular type), the cardiovascular effects increase with gestational age and may be life threatening. During pregnancy, maternal blood volume increases by 40 %, resulting in a 30–50 % increase in cardiac output. In Marfan syndrome it is generally accepted that a pregnancy is contraindicated when the aortic diameter exceeds 50 mm. Likewise, patients affected with EDS type IV are at increased risk of arterial, bowel and uterine rupture. The condition has one of the highest mortality rates for pregnant women with significant morbidity being common if the mother survives. Although not reported, one may assume that ovum pick-up in EDS IV women also be risky. Counselling against PGD treatment and pregnancy due to the high complication rates could be advocated in certain cases.

In Duchenne/Becker muscular dystrophy carrier women may show progressive dilated cardiomyopathy, leading to a decreased left ventricular ejection fraction and congestive heart failure. Women affected with myotonic dystrophy type 1 may be faced with cardiac rhythm disturbances, with an increased risk of sudden death. Thus, preconceptional cardiac evaluation prior to PGD treatment and surveillance during pregnancy are recommended. Other neuromuscular disorders may also be complicated by cardiac involvement, such as the laminopathies and different types of limb girdle muscular dystrophy.

Disorders of Haemostasis

Carriers of inherited bleeding disorders may face several haemostatic challenges during PGD treatment and pregnancy. Haemophilias A and B are one of the most prevalent indications for PGD and are both inherited as X-linked disorders. Before starting PGD treatment, female haemophilia carriers should have their factor VIII/IX levels checked to assess the need for prophylactic treatment during oocyte retrieval. One must also be aware of possible bleeding complications after the intervention, so prolonged surveillance is recommended. In haemophilia A, administration of DDAVP may give temporary increase in factor VIII level, while in haemophilia B, administration of recombinant factor IX may be indicated.

Skeletal Disorders

In women with achondroplasia, difficulties in ovarian stimulation and oocyte retrieval have been reported. Due to abnormal pelvic position of the ovaries, oocyte retrieval could be difficult even under general anaesthesia. Vaginal delivery may be complicated in affected women due to pelvic skeletal abnormalities, and a planned caesarean section may be advisable.

Conditions with Tumour Formation Potential or Increased Risk of Malignancy

Tuberous sclerosis complex type 1 or 2 (TSC 1 or 2) is characterised by skin, brain, kidney (angiomyolipomas, renal cysts, renal cell carcinomas), heart (rhabdomyomas, arrhythmias) and lung (lymphangioleiomyomatosis) involvement. Calcifications of the ovaries may hinder oocyte retrieval. Renal angiomyolipoma carries the risk of growth and rupture in pregnancy. Evaluation of affected organs may reveal abnormalities that may interfere with safe PGD treatment.

Familial Adenomatous Polyposis Coli

Women suffering from familial adenomatous polyposis coli (FAP) are confronted with hundreds to thousands of precancerous colonic polyps, beginning in puberty. Without colectomy, colon cancer is inevitable. Extraintestinal manifestations, such as intra-abdominal desmoids tumours, may also be present. Most patients undergo a colectomy with ileal pouch-anal anastomosis at young adult age, frequently rendering oocyte retrieval more difficult due to post-operative distortion of pelvic anatomy.

Could the Course of the Genetic Condition Be Affected by PGD Treatment or Pregnancy?

In general, there is no evidence that PGD treatment affects the course of genetic disease. Hormonal stimulation for PGD treatment could be a concern in BRCA mutation carriers. Long-term and more extensive studies on ART-related risks for BRCA patients are needed.

Key Points
- In PGD patients, careful preconceptional assessment, often by a multidisciplinary team, is paramount.
- Special consideration is given to gynaecological pathology relevant to the underlying genetic condition.
- Carrier state of some genetic conditions may be associated with subfertility and require specific intervention during PGD treatment.
- Medical challenges encountered secondary to the underlying genetic condition should be managed via a personalised treatment plan, avoidance of multiple pregnancy and close surveillance during pregnancy.
- PGD treatment does not alter the disease state of affected patients; however large follow-up studies are needed.

Further Reading

Azim A, Costantini-Ferrando M, Lostritto K, Oktay K. Relative potencies of anastrozole and letrozole to suppress estradiol in breast cancer patients undergoing ovarian stimulation before in vitro fertilization. J Clin Endocrinol Metab. 2007;92:2197–200.

Chen SH, Escudero T, Cekleniak NA, Sable DB, Garrisi MG, Munne S. Patterns of ovarian response to gonadotropin stimulation in female carriers of balanced translocation. Fertil Seril. 2005;83:1504–9.

Claustres M, Guittard C, Bozon D, Chevalier F, Verlingue C, Ferec C, Girodon E, Cazeneuve C, Bienvenu T, Lalau G, et al. Spectrum of CFTR mutations in cystic fibrosis and in congenital absence of the vas deferens in France. Hum Mutat. 2000;16:143–56.

Dechanet C, Castelli C, Reyftmann L, Coubes C, Hamamah S, Hedon B, Dechaud H, Anahory T. Myotonic dystrophy type 1 and PGD: ovarian stimulation response and correlation analysis between ovarian reserve and genotype. RBM Online. 2010;20:610–8.

Donnelly RT, Pinto NM, Kocolas I, Yetman AT. The immediate and long-term impact of pregnancy on aortic growth rate and mortality in women with Marfan syndrome. J Am Coll Cardiol. 2012;60:224–9.

Hammond R, Oligbo N. Ehlers Danlos syndrome type IV and pregnancy. Arch Gynecol Obstet. 2012;285:51–4.

Hermans MC, Pinto YM, Merkies IS, de Die-Smulders CE, Crijns HJ, Faber CG. Hereditary muscular dystrophies and the heart. Neuromuscul Disord. 2010;20:479–92.

Kotsopoulos J, Librach CL, Lubinski J, Gronwald J, Kim-Sing C, Ghadirian P, Lynch HT, Moller P, Foulkes WD, Randall S, Manoukian S, Pasini B, Tung N, Ainsworth PJ, Cummings S, Sun P, Narod SA, Hereditary Breast Cancer Clinical Study Group. Infertility, treatment of infertility, and the risk of breast cancer among women with BRCA1 and BRCA2 mutations: a case-control study. Cancer Causes Control. 2008;19:1111–9.

Moutou C, Rongieres C, Bettahar-Lebugle K, Gardes N, Phillippe C, Viville S. Preimplantation genetic diagnosis for achondroplasia: genetics and gynaecological limits and difficulties. Hum Reprod. 2003;18:509–14.

Oktay K, et al. Association of BRCA1 mutations with occult primary ovarian insufficiency: a possible explanation for the link between infertility and breast/ovarian cancer risks. J Clin Oncol. 2010; 28:240–4.

Platteau P, Sermon K, Seneca S, Van Steirteghem A, Devroey P, Liebaers I. Preimplantation genetic diagnosis for fragile Xa syndrome: difficult but not impossible. Hum Reprod. 2002;17:2807–12.

Sarkar PS, Paul S, Han J, Reddy S. Six5 is required for spermatogenic cell survival and spermiogenesis. Hum Mol Genet. 2004;13:1421–31.

Schlessinger D, Herrera L, Crisponi L, Mumm S, Percsepe A, Pelligrini M, et al. Genes and translocations involved in POF. Am J Med Genet. 2002;111:328–33.

Thornhill AR, deDie-Smulders CE, Geraedts JP, Harper JC, Harton GL, Lavery SA, Mouto C, Robinson MD, Schmutzler AG, Scriven PN, Sermon KD. ESHRE PGD consortium 'best practice guidelines for clinical preimplantation genetic diagnosis (PGD) and preimplantation genetic screening (PGS)'. Hum Reprod. 2004;20:35–48.

Verpoest W, De Rademaeker M, Sermon K, et al. Real and expected delivery rates of patients with myotonic dystrophy undergoing intracytoplasmic sperm injection and preimplantation genetic diagnosis. Hum Reprod. 2008;23:1654–60.

Zreik TG, Mazloom A, Chen Y, Vannucci M, Pinnix CC, Fulton S, et al. Fertility drugs and the risk of breast cancer: a meta-analysis and review. Breast Cancer Res Treat. 2010;124:13–26.

Chapter 6
Embryology and PGD

Virginia N. Bolton

The Role of the Clinical Embryologist in PGD

Preimplantation genetic diagnosis (PGD) was first postulated as having potential for clinical application in 1965. However, the technical difficulties of sampling the preimplantation embryo, providing sufficient material and sufficient time for genetic analysis before embryo transfer, meant that successful realisation of this vision was not achieved for a further 22 years.

The pivotal role of the clinical embryologist in PGD is in minimising damage to embryos throughout the procedures that are necessary for the technique: in providing an environment for the routine fertilisation of oocytes and culture of resulting human preimplantation embryos; in the technical expertise enabling biopsy of embryos at whichever stage is deemed appropriate; in performing the biopsy procedure in an environment where DNA or adventitious agent contamination is minimised; in collecting biopsied cells using methods that minimise the risk of loss, contamination or mismatch

V.N. Bolton, MA, PhD
Assisted Conception Unit and PGD Centre, Guy's and St. Thomas'
Hospital NHS Foundation Trust, 11th Floor, Tower Wing,
Guy's Hospital, Great Maze Pond, London SE1 9RT, UK
e-mail: virginia.bolton@gstt.nhs.uk

T. El-Toukhy, P. Braude (eds.), *Preimplantation Genetic
Diagnosis in Clinical Practice*, DOI 10.1007/978-1-4471-2948-6_6,
© Springer-Verlag London 2014

between each embryo and its diagnosis; and in the successful cryopreservation of embryos, whether whilst awaiting results of the genetic diagnosis or for storage of unaffected embryos surplus to those transferred in a fresh cycle of treatment.

Fertilisation Methods

Where male fertility is not in doubt, and where genetic analysis of chromosomal disorders is to be undertaken using fluorescence in situ hybridisation (FISH), fertilisation may be achieved using conventional in vitro fertilisation (IVF), with insemination and overnight incubation of oocytes with prepared spermatozoa. In such cases, any residual cumulus cells that may remain adhered to and additional spermatozoa that may be bound to the *zona pellucida* (ZP, see Chap. 8) of the developing embryo will not impact upon the diagnostic test that is undertaken. However, if a molecular diagnostic technique is required, such as in the diagnosis of a single-gene disorder, additional steps must be taken to remove the risk of contamination with maternal or paternal DNA. Thus, the use of intracytoplasmic sperm injection (ICSI), where maternal cumulus cells are removed from the ZP before injection of a single spermatozoon to achieve fertilisation, is essential for all cases where PGD of single-gene disorders is to be undertaken; furthermore, any cumulus cells still adhering to the zona pellucida must be removed before biopsy.

Biopsy Procedures

Breaching the Zona Pellucida

Techniques for breaching the zona pellucida (ZP) were developed for the biopsy of blastomeres from cleavage stage embryos and include chemical drilling using acid Tyrode's or pronase solution, partial zona dissection (PZD) and laser ablation. Each has the potential to damage the embryo, whether by exposure to the chemical agent used or through mechanical damage, and none has been shown unequivocally to be the method of choice. Indeed, no difference has been demonstrated between any of the techniques, in terms of the effect on implantation rates of manipulated embryos, when used for assisted hatching during cleavage. However, it has been recommended that mechanical, rather than chemical or laser, drilling should be used for polar body biopsy of oocytes because of the sensitivity of the meiotic spindle to damage, where care must be taken to minimise exposure of the embryo to reduced pH.

Adaptations of the original mechanical PZD method include the use of a piezo-micromanipulator, in which a piezoelectric pulse induces a vibratory motion in the dissecting needle; 3-dimensional PZD (3D-PZD), where the microneedle is used to make a cross-shaped breach in the ZP; and long zona dissection, where a long slit is made in the ZP using a modified holding pipette (LZD).

Whilst zona drilling using a laser is technically more straightforward than chemical techniques, and there are reports that laser drilling does not impair embryonic development to the blastocyst stage and implantation, its use is not without the potential to harm embryos.

Selection of a given method may be based on practical and economic considerations, including whether it is to be used for polar body biopsy, cleavage stage blastomere biopsy (Fig. 6.1) or trophectoderm biopsy of blastocyst stage embryos.

With all methods for zona breaching, the embryo is placed in a droplet of medium, usually buffered for use in air (HEPES or MOPS buffer) under oil on a warmed microscope stage. For cleavage stage biopsy, the medium used is free of Ca^{2+} and Mg^+, in order to reduce blastomere adhesion and facilitate removal of a single cell. The embryo is secured using a gentle vacuum applied to a holding pipette; once an opening has been generated in the ZP, cell(s) is aspirated through the breach in the ZP using the biopsy pipette (outer diameter 50 μm; inner diameter 35 μm).

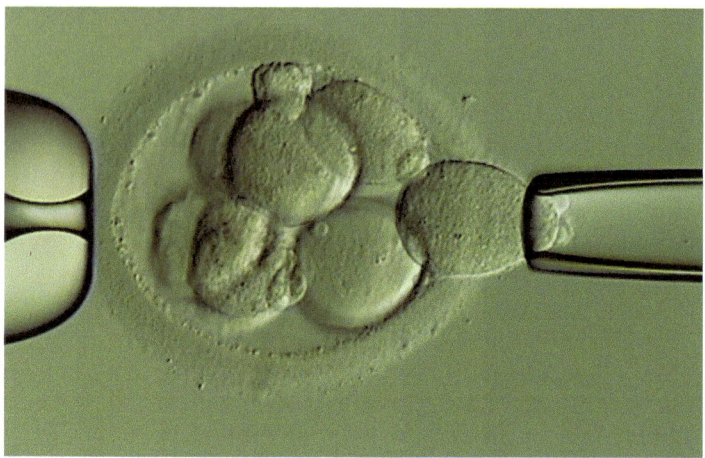

FIGURE 6.1 Stereophotomicrograph of a day 3 cleavage stage human embryo on a glass holding pipette, with a single blastomere being extracted through the hole breached in the zona pellucida. Note the intact nucleus in the cell being removed

The apparatus and micropipettes used for chemical drilling are shown in Figs. 6.1a and 6.2b. With this technique, a small hole is created in the ZP by controlled application of a stream of acid Tyrode's (or pronase) solution, expelled from the drilling pipette (inner diameter 5–6 μm).

For PZD, the embryo is secured with a holding pipette as with chemical drilling, and a slit is made in the ZP by rubbing a PZD pipette against the holding pipette with a sawing motion. The immobilised embryo may be squeezed with a biopsy pipette until a blastomere of a cleavage stage embryo is extruded, followed by aspiration with a biopsy pipette, or cell(s) may be aspirated as described for chemical drilling.

For laser ablation, the apparatus for which is shown in Fig. 6.3, the ZP of the secured embryo is breached, taking care with blastocyst stage embryos to orientate the embryo so that the breach is made in a region away from the inner cell mass (ICM), with aspirated trophectoderm cells excised using the laser.

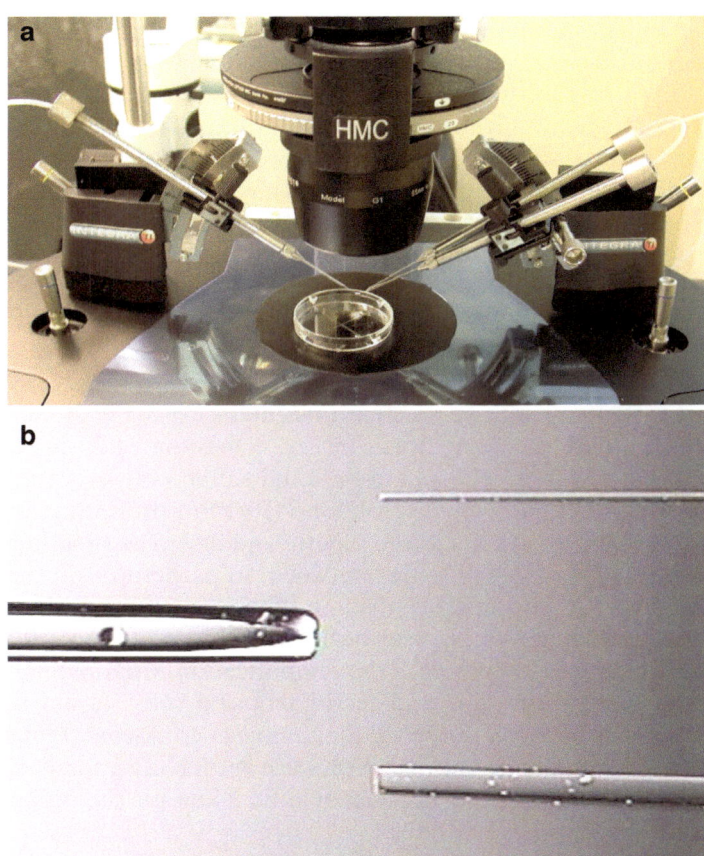

FIGURE 6.2 Micromanipulation apparatus for chemical zona drilling. (a) Micromanipulators attached to an inverted phase microscope, showing the attachments for the holding pipette (*left*) and drilling and biopsy pipettes (*right*). (b) Micropipettes used for holding (*left*), drilling (*upper right*) and biopsy (*lower right*)

Handling Biopsied Material

When required for processing for molecular analysis, precautions must be taken to prevent DNA contamination; when biopsied cells are to be processed for chromosome analysis, such precautions may be less stringent. Biopsies should be carried out using sterile equipment in a minimum Class I flow hood, which provides material with protection from airborne contamination throughout the procedure, and the practitioner processing the biopsied cells should wear protective clothing (hairnet, facemask, theatre gown and sterile gloves) that must be changed if any contact is made with potential sources of contamination.

Biopsied cells must be rinsed thoroughly to ensure removal of all potential contaminants, but with care to avoid causing cell lysis, which may compromise the chance of yielding results. In practice, this entails rinsing in at least 3 sequential drops of wash buffer, consisting of a simple solution such as phosphate-buffered saline (PBS) supplemented with polyvinylpyrrolidone (PVP) to prevent adhesion of biopsied cells to the pipette and dish. The pipette is rinsed in fresh wash buffer between drops, before transfer of the cells into microcentrifuge tubes containing PBS, in no more than 1–2 μl wash buffer to avoid dilution of the reagents used for lysis and DNA amplification. Micropipettes used for rinsing and transfer of biopsied cells should be changed between samples to minimise cross-contamination. A sample of the stock of wash buffer used for each series of biopsy procedures should be taken for the preparation of a negative control.

Embryo Development

Biopsied embryos are rinsed through fresh drops of warmed culture medium before being returned to culture. This is particularly important when chemical drilling has been used and for cleavage stage biopsies where Ca^{2+}- and Mg^+-free medium will have been used, in order to remove traces of the chemical agent, biopsy medium and HEPES or MOPS buffer from the culture medium.

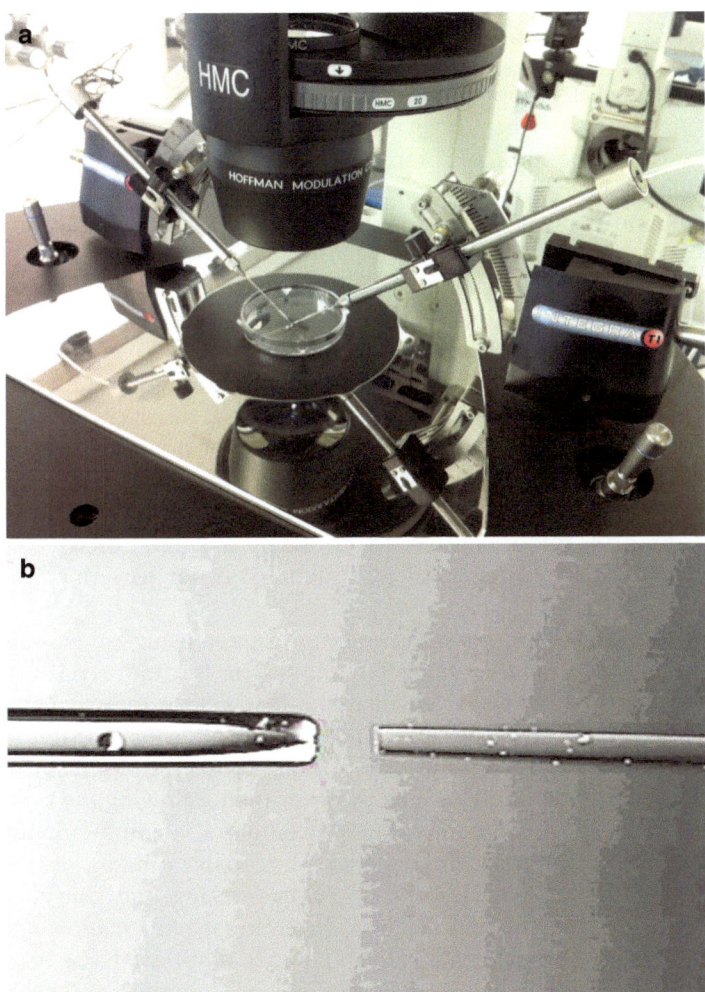

FIGURE 6.3 Micromanipulation apparatus for laser ablation. (**a**) Micromanipulators attached to an inverted phase microscope, showing the attachments for the holding pipette (*left*) and biopsy pipette (*right*). (**b**) Micropipettes used for holding (*left*) and biopsy (*right*)

Cryopreservation of Biopsied Embryos

Successful cryopreservation is an essential component of any PGD service, for several reasons. First, it may be necessary, on occasion, for biopsied embryos to be cryopreserved whilst allowing sufficient time for the results of genetic diagnosis of the biopsied material to become available; second, embryos found to be free of the genetic disorder under investigation, surplus to the fresh embryo(s) transferred in the initial treatment cycle and that appear morphologically to be developing normally, should be cryopreserved in order to increase the chance, and the number, of successful pregnancies following a single IVF/ICSI cycle; third, cryopreservation increases the cost-effectiveness of a single cycle of IVF/ICSI and PGD, both in terms of financial and emotional investment; and, finally, successful cryopreservation supports the incentive to transfer a single unaffected embryo in each cycle of treatment, in order to reduce the risk of multiple pregnancy.

Biopsied embryos may be cryopreserved using either long-established slow-freezing techniques or the more recently adopted technique of vitrification. It has been reported that implantation and successful pregnancy following transfer of slow-frozen and thawed embryos following blastomere biopsy at the cleavage stage is lower than following the same procedures carried out with intact embryos, possibly because of increased vulnerability to the toxic effects of the cryoprotectant reagents used in slow freezing when the zona pellucida has been breached. In contrast, vitrification and warming of both biopsied and intact embryos have been reported to yield equivalent survival, implantation and pregnancy rates. For this reason, vitrification may be the preferred method for cryopreservation following embryo biopsy.

With advances in the understanding of the culture requirements of human embryos, and the availability of media that support the development of embryos to the blastocyst stage in vitro, successful cryopreservation of embryos surplus to those transferred fresh may be carried out routinely on days 5 and 6 of development, whether biopsy takes place during cleavage or at the blastocyst stage, once the results of genetic diagnosis are available. An alternative approach that allows genetic analysis to be undertaken with less time constraints is to vitrify all biopsied blastocysts immediately post-biopsy whilst awaiting the results of diagnosis and discarding those found to be affected once the results are known.

Documentation and Safety

It is essential that the result of genetic diagnosis specific for each embryo is reliable and specific to that embryo, and rigorous measures must be implemented to remove any risk of ambiguity. Embryos must be cultured after biopsy using a method that will ensure their accurate identification; culture in separate dishes, or culture in dishes with moulded, numbered wells that ensure embryo identification and segregation is mandatory. The cells biopsied from each embryo must be processed using corresponding labelling between cells and embryo, with clear documentation and witnessed processing steps to ensure that the genetic diagnosis for each embryo is matched unambiguously to the biopsied material from which the diagnosis is made.

Key Points
- The success of any PGD programme relies on there being a successful embryology laboratory for assisted conception.
- The method for breaching the zona pellucida may be selected according to practical and financial considerations.

- Rigorous measures must be implemented to eliminate all possible sources of contamination of biopsied material, including the use of ICSI for molecular diagnostic cases.
- Rigorous measures must be implemented to ensure segregation and accurate identification of individual embryos and the cells biopsied from them.
- A successful cryopreservation programme is essential to provide the maximum possible success rate for a PGD service.

Further Reading

Harton GL, Magli MC, Lundin K, Montag M, Lemmen J, Harper JC, et al. ESHRE PGD Consortium/Embryology Special Interest Group: best practice guidelines for polar body and embryo biopsy for preimplantation genetic diagnosis/screening (PGD/PGS). Hum Reprod. 2011;26:41–6.

Chapter 7
PGD for Sex Determination and Chromosome Rearrangements: FISH and Emerging Technologies

Paul N. Scriven and Caroline Mackie Ogilvie

Fluorescence in situ hybridisation (FISH) on the fixed nuclei of biopsied blastomeres from day 3 cleavage-stage embryos using target-specific DNA probes has been for over a decade the technique of choice for detecting chromosome imbalance in embryos from couples referred for PGD because of a chromosome rearrangement. It has also been used to select female embryos in families with the rare X-linked diseases for which a mutation-specific test was not available or practical.

P.N. Scriven, BSc, PhD (✉)
Medical & Molecular Genetics, King's College London
Medical School, Cytogenetics, 5th Floor Tower Wing,
Guy's Hospital, Great Maze Pond, London SE1 9RT, UK
e-mail: paul.scriven@kcl.ac.uk

C. Mackie Ogilvie, BSc, DPhil
Cytogenetics Department, Guy's and St. Thomas' Hospital NHS
Foundation Trust, 5th Floor, Tower Wing, Guy's Hospital,
Great Maze Pond, London SE1 9RT, UK
e-mail: caroline.ogilvie@genetics.kcl.ac.uk

T. El-Toukhy, P. Braude (eds.), *Preimplantation Genetic Diagnosis in Clinical Practice*, DOI 10.1007/978-1-4471-2948-6_7, © Springer-Verlag London 2014

Sex Determination Using FISH

PGD for sex-linked diseases, using FISH to differentiate between male and female embryos followed by the transfer of female embryos, is usually offered where the specific mutation associated with the condition is not known or is associated with more than one gene on the X chromosome (for instance, a strong family history of males with mental retardation) or where a specific test for a mutation is not available (rare conditions, such as choroideremia). In most cases, the defective gene on the X chromosome tends to have little or no phenotypic effect on carrier females because there is a second normal copy of the gene on the other X chromosome, whereas males with only a single X chromosome carrying the defective gene are affected with the disease.

The major disadvantage of using FISH for sexing is that it does not differentiate between a normal male and an affected male embryo, which restricts the number of embryos available for transfer and excludes the possibility of a male child. It also doesn't differentiate between normal and "carrier" female embryos, which may result in heterozygous females with mild clinical features of the sex-linked condition (such as haemophilia), due to skewed X-inactivation of the normal allele.

Test Design

Figure 7.1 shows the results from a FISH test containing one probe specific for each centromere region of the X (green) and Y (red) chromosomes and one autosome (to determine the ploidy of the nucleus), hybridised to a single blastomere nucleus, showing a male chromosome complement. Using this test, scoring errors due to probe binding failure or signal splitting or overlapping (co-localisation) could result in inaccurate test results. However, in order to misdiagnose a male embryo as a female, two errors are required: failure to detect the red Y chromosome signal and inaccurately scoring one green X signal as two (Fig. 7.2). Diagnosis using only one biopsied cell with a clearly visible single nucleus is therefore a robust test for determining the sex of an embryo.

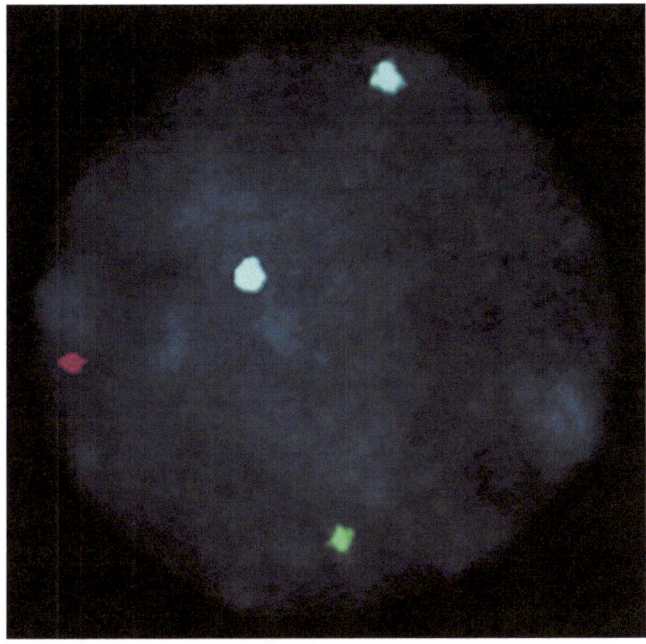

FigURE 7.1 Single-cell nucleus hybridised with FISH probes for the centromere regions of chromosomes X (*green*), Y (*red*) and 18 (*blue*), showing a normal male chromosome complement

On average, only 30 % of embryos tested have a transferable (female) test result using this strategy. This is less than the theoretical expectation of 50 % due to a combination of factors, which include multinucleated cells, FISH signal scoring error (only one scoring error will exclude a normal female embryo), chromosome aneuploidy and test failure (Fig. 7.3).

PGD for Chromosome Rearrangements Using FISH

The most common chromosome rearrangements are reciprocal translocations (1 in 500 individuals) and Robertsonian translocations (1 in 1,000 individuals). Couples carrying a chromosome rearrangement usually present with a variety of

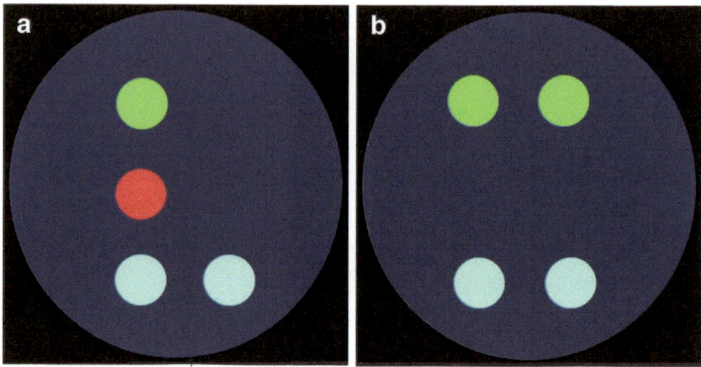

FIGURE 7.2 Cartoon of expected patterns for (**a**) a normal male cell, and (**b**) a normal female cell, using the FISH probes as in Fig. 7.1. Misdiagnosis of a male cell (**a**) as female (**b**) would require failure to detect the red signal and erroneous detection of an extra green signal

difficult obstetric histories, including live-born offspring with congenital abnormalities due to chromosome imbalance, termination of affected pregnancies and recurrent miscarriage where a direct association with an abnormal karyotype has not been established. Most fertile translocation couples have an excellent chance of a successful outcome by natural conception within a realistic timeframe, and these couples should therefore be carefully counselled prior to embarking on a PGD cycle.

Reciprocal Translocation

Reciprocal translocations are typically a terminal exchange between two different chromosomes with no loss of genetic material (balanced) (see Fig. 7.4) and hence no phenotypic consequences for carriers. Assuming one breakpoint per chromosome band, there are approximately 250,000 different possible permutations, which means that most reciprocal translocations are unique to each family. At meiosis, segregation results in gametes with between zero and three copies of

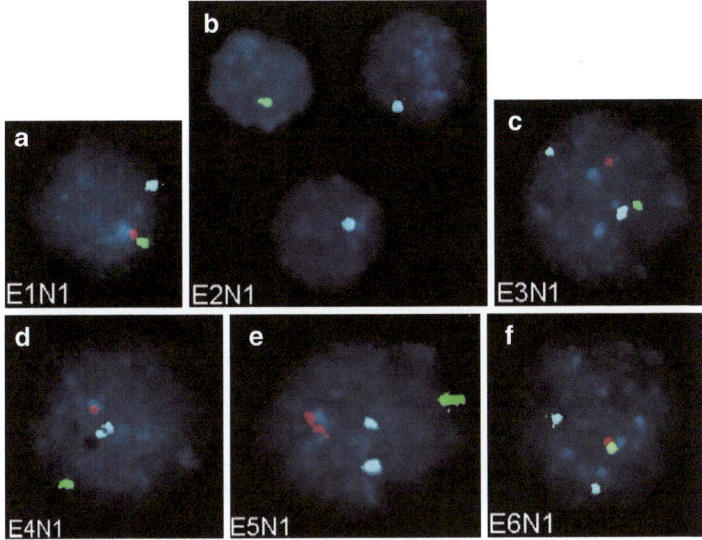

FIGURE 7.3 Single-cell nuclei from a PGD cycle for X-linked disease hybridised with FISH probes as in Fig. 7.1. Six embryos were tested, of which four (**c**, **d**, **e** and **f**) showed a normal male signal pattern, whilst one (**a**) showed an abnormal male signal pattern (only one *blue* chromosome 18 signal), and one (**b**) showed multinucleation, with signal patterns indicating the presence on only a single sex chromosome. No embryos were therefore available for transfer

the four translocation segments (two centric segments containing the centromeres and the two exchanged segments) and embryos with between one and four copies. There are 32 theoretically possible outcomes from meiotic segregation of reciprocal translocation: normal and balanced products (with two copies of each segment) and 30 unbalanced products with different permutations that deviate from two copies of each segment.

Depending on the chromosomes involved and the breakpoints, the risk of a live-born child with an unbalanced translocation ranges from <1 % up to 30 %. The risk of spontaneous miscarriage is typically in the region of 20–30 % compared to the general population background risk of 10–15 %.

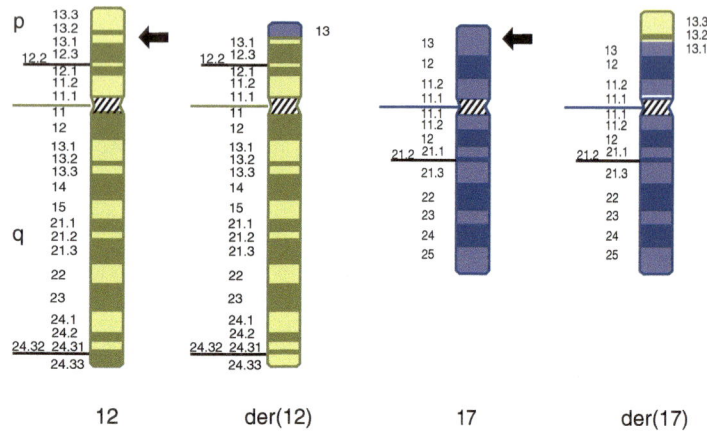

FIGURE 7.4 Cartoon representation of a reciprocal translocation between chromosomes 12 (represented in *yellow*) and chromosome 17 (represented in *blue*). *Arrows* show the breakpoints of the translocation

Robertsonian Translocations

Robertsonian translocations are the result of the centric fusion of two "acrocentric" chromosomes thus producing a large derivative chromosome (der). This results in a chromosome count of 45, but with no loss of active genetic material (Fig. 7.5). However, the presence of the translocation may result in meiotic arrest, leading to oligozoospermia in some balanced male carriers. Abnormal meiotic segregation of these translocations results in gametes with nullisomy or disomy for one of the chromosomes involved in the rearrangement and consequently to an embryo with monosomy or trisomy for one of the chromosomes involved. Monosomy for these chromosomes is not compatible with life, and most translocation trisomy conceptuses are expected to result in first-trimester loss. Thus, the risk of spontaneous miscarriage for carriers of Robertsonian translocations may be increased compared to the general population background risk of 10–15 %.

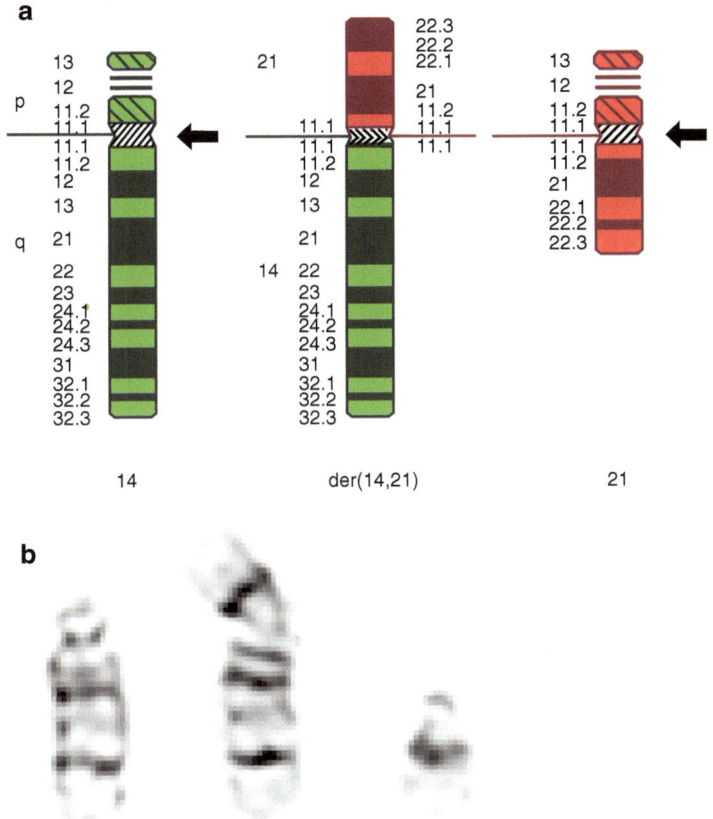

FIGURE 7.5 (**a**) Cartoon representation of a Robertsonian translocation between chromosomes 14 (represented in *green*) and 21 (represented in *red*). (**b**) The same Robertsonian translocation chromosomes as seen at 1,000× magnification following mitotic arrest, enzyme digestion and staining

The most common Robertsonian translocation is between chromosomes 13 and 14; trisomy for chromosome 13 results in Patau syndrome. Carriers have an empirical risk of approximately 1 % of trisomy 13 or uniparental disomy for chromosome 14 at second-trimester prenatal diagnosis (rescue of trisomy or monosomy 14 can result in two copies of chromosome 14 from the same parent). This is consistent with our experience that 7 and 2 % of embryos have trisomy 13 for female and male carriers, respectively.

The next most common Robertsonian translocation is between chromosomes 14 and 21 (Fig. 7.5); trisomy 21 results in Down syndrome. Female carriers have a 15 % risk of trisomy 21 at amniocentesis and 10 % at term. However, for male carriers, the risk of trisomy 21 is less than 1 %. This is consistent with our experience that 22 % and 0 % of embryos from female and male carriers, respectively, have trisomy 21.

Test Design and Patient Workup

The recommended practice for all chromosome rearrangements is that the test should include sufficient probes to detect all the unbalanced segregation products of the rearrangement and, if testing only one cell, to have two probes that are diagnostic for any chromosome imbalance that has potential to be viable or that is associated with segregation products that are likely to be frequent.

Once the test has been designed, probe mixes should be tested on cells from the translocation carrier to ensure the probes selected hybridise as expected and are informative for the translocation segments. Cells are also analysed from the noncarrier partner to ensure that the probes hybridise normally. Interphase nuclei are scored to make a quantitative assessment of the assay and a qualitative assessment of FISH signal intensity and discreteness. These assays only detect copy number and cannot differentiate between normal and rearranged but balanced chromosomes.

Robertsonian Translocations

Our PGD tests include two FISH probes for chromosomes 13 and 21 in cases where the rearrangement involves either or both of these chromosomes (see Fig. 7.6), as trisomy for

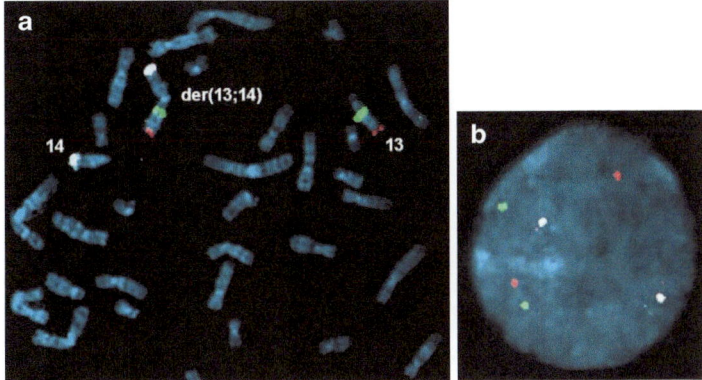

FIGURE 7.6 (**a**) FISH probes for the long arms of chromosomes 13 (*red* and *green*) and 14 (*white*), hybridised to condensed, stained chromosomes (visualised by fluorescence microscopy), from a carrier of a Robertsonian translocation between chromosomes 13 and 14. (**b**) Nondividing single-cell nucleus from the same preparation

either of these chromosomes may be viable. In our experience for Robertsonian translocations, 48 % of embryos tested have a transferable test result consistent with a normal or balanced complement for the translocation chromosomes.

Two-Way Terminal Reciprocal Translocations

At least three FISH probes, one each for three of the four segments, are required to detect all the different theoretical meiotic segregation products resulting in sperm or eggs with chromosome imbalance. At Guy's PGD Centre, we recommend using a probe for each of the translocated segments and a third probe for the centric segment of the smallest chromosome, each labelled with a different fluorochrome and visualised with appropriate filters (three-colour FISH). It is critical to assess the nature of the chromosome rearrangement prior to designing preimplantation genetic FISH tests; failure to do so could result in a significant risk of an affected pregnancy. In our experience for reciprocal

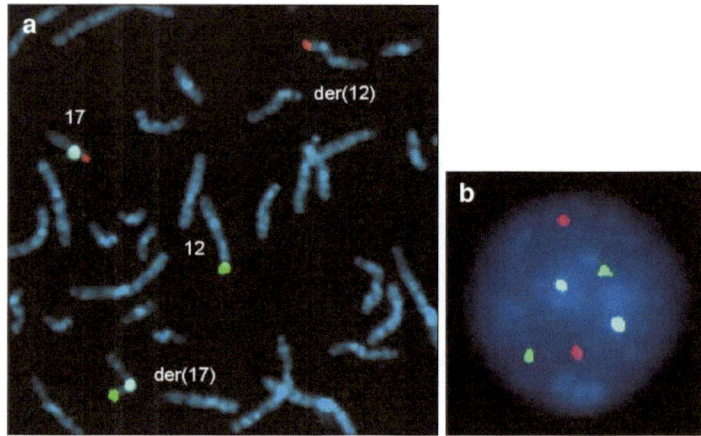

FIGURE 7.7 (**a**) FISH probes for the short arm terminal regions of chromosomes 12 (*green*) and 17 (*red*) and the centromere region of chromosome 17 (*blue*) hybridised to condensed, stained chromosomes (visualised by fluorescence microscopy), from a carrier of the translocation shown in Fig. 7.4. (**b**) Nondividing single-cell nucleus from the same preparation

translocations, only 22 % of embryos tested have a transferable test result.

Figure 7.7 shows a peripheral blood metaphase spread and an interphase nucleus from the carrier partner hybridised with FISH probes for the translocation shown in Fig. 7.4; green and red FISH probes specific for the short arm subtelomere regions of chromosomes 12 and 17 and a blue FISH probe specific for the centromere region of chromosome 17 show two copies of each region.

A Decade's Experience Using FISH at Guy's and St Thomas' Centre for PGD

Table 7.1 shows the number of cycles started and the clinical outcome. Table 7.2 shows diagnostic accuracy measures using FISH. In experienced hands the accuracy of PGD testing two

TABLE 7.1 Clinical outcome for PGD using FISH tests for sex determination for sex-linked diseases and chromosome rearrangements

	Sex determination	Reciprocal translocations	Robertsonian translocations
Couples started	51	59	28
Biopsy cycles	71	110	42
Live birth deliveries	24	26	15
Children born	32	32	20
Clinical pregnancy losses (%)	4	10	12
Live births/ biopsy (%)	34	24	36
Live births/ couple (%)	47	36	54
Cumulative/couple (3 cycles) (%)	67	51	76

chromosome pairs using the FISH technique is high, and the risk of an affected pregnancy following PGD using a well-designed test is low. The risk of spontaneous miscarriage following PGD for translocations is likely to be reduced at least to that observed in the general population.

Emerging Technologies

Polymerase Chain Reaction Microsatellite Analysis

PCR analysis using short tandem repeat (STR) microsatellite DNA markers may offer some improvement over the FISH technique. In addition to identifying copy number of translocation segments, it will also detect clinically relevant uniparental disomy (UPD), such as UPD 14, which can arise following "rescue" of Robertsonian translocation trisomy 14, resulting in a balanced chromosome complement but with both remaining homologues of chromosome 14 originating from one parent (Fig. 7.8).

TABLE 7.2 PGD test performance

Diagnostic measure	Sex determination	Reciprocal translocations	Robertsonian translocations	
			Female	Male
Specificity %	84	75	80	70
Sensitivity %	100	100	100	100
Accuracy %	94	92	89	78
Prevalence %	60	67	43	28
PPV %	91	89	79	57
NPV %	100	100	100	100
False abnormal %	6	8	11	22
False normal %	0	0	0	0

Sensitivity, specificity and positive (PPV) and negative (NPV) predictive value are the most useful indicators of diagnostic performance. Sensitivity and specificity give a measure of the quality of the test; positive and negative predictive accuracy give measures of the effect that different practical situations have on the test and give the posttest probability of being affected or unaffected. Confirmation of diagnosis studies, where embryos not transferred or frozen are spread and the remaining cells analysed and compared to the result from the biopsied cell, can be used to estimate the analytical performance of the preimplantation test. The false normal and abnormal rates are calculated as a proportion of the total test results (test perspective not outcome perspective)

The limitations of using PCR for chromosomal rearrangements include:

1. Extensive workup may be necessary to find sufficient informative STR markers for all the translocation segments; however, development of generic STR multiplexes for chromosome ends can circumvent this problem.
2. The technique might not be suitable for translocations with breakpoints near the telomeres because of the uncertainty of the location of the STR markers in relation to the breakpoints.

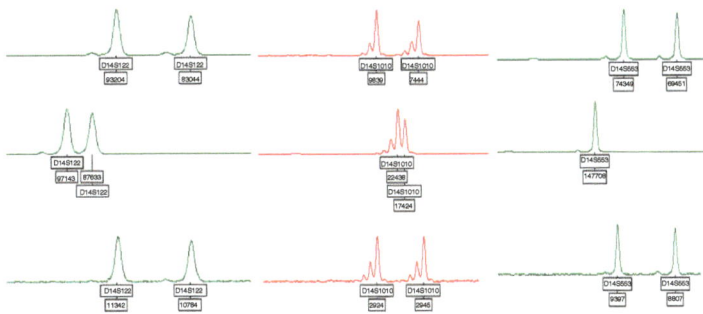

FIGURE 7.8 Electrophoretic traces showing amplified microsatellite regions (D14S1434 and D14S127) on chromosome 14 from an embryo *top row* and the same regions in both parents *middle and bottom row*. Pairs of electrophoretic peaks demonstrate the presence of two copies of chromosome 14; comparison of peak positions on the electrophoretogram shows that the embryo has inherited both copies of chromosome 14 from one parent

Microarray Analysis

Array comparative genomic hybridisation (aCGH) and single nucleotide polymorphism (SNP) microarray have the potential benefit of testing for imbalance arising from complex chromosome rearrangements (involving more than two chromosomes) and can also be used to screen for aneuploidy of chromosomes not involved in the chromosome rearrangement (24-chromosome analysis). Additionally, the preclinical workup associated with FISH and PCR methodology is not required, and the analysis can include every chromosome and is more amenable to automation. Whole-genome amplification (WGA) is required for PGD using microarrays, since a single nucleus contains only ~6 pg of DNA.

Array CGH

Array CGH uses oligonucleotide probes or DNA segments from bacterial artificial chromosomes (BACs), of known size and location in the genome. These DNA segments

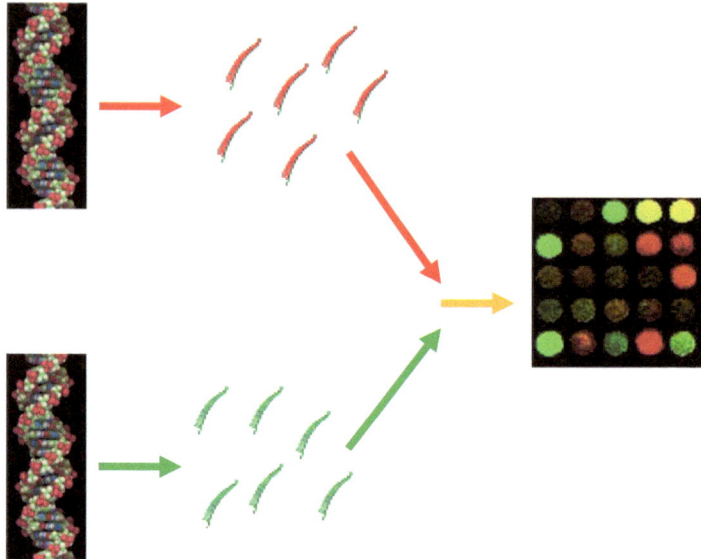

FIGURE 7.9 Cartoon representation of principle of array CGH. Total genomic DNA from test material is prepared as small fragments and labelled with a red fluorochrome, then mixed with reference DNA similarly prepared, and labelled with a green fluorochrome. The mixed pool of DNA is added to the array slide, where sequences compete for complementary sequences on the slide. The resulting fluorescence ratios give information on the relative copy number of each sequence

are attached to a glass slide, and the DNA from the test sample and a normal male reference sample is labelled with different fluorophores and hybridised to the probes on the slide (Fig. 7.9). The fluorescence intensity ratio of the test and the reference DNA is measured, to identify copy number changes (gain or loss) for a particular location in the genome.

The limitations of aCGH include:

1. It is not possible to differentiate a normal 46,XX (diploid) euploid chromosome complement from abnormal complements such as 23,X (haploid), 69,XXX (triploid) and 92,XXXX (tetraploid).

2. It may not be possible to test rearrangements with very terminal breakpoints (see above).
3. Some aCGH studies have found a high degree of chromosome instability with small regions of segmental gain and loss where the clinical significance is uncertain.

SNP Microarrays

SNP microarrays use similar technology, but the oligonucleotide probes are specific for regions containing single nucleotide polymorphisms (SNPs) and therefore have the additional advantage of detecting regions of loss of heterozygosity. If parental SNP genotypes are known, the analysis can also differentiate haploidy, triploidy and diploidy (but not tetraploidy), detect clinically relevant UPD and differentiate meiotic and mitotic chromosome trisomy (meiotic trisomy will have been present at conception but mitotic trisomy must be post-zygotic and due to mosaicism might not be representative of the whole embryo).

Key Points
- FISH testing to identify the sex of the embryos in cases of X-linked disease is robust and reliable, but normal male embryos will be discarded.
- Reciprocal translocations are generally unique; individual tests should be designed for each couple following assessment of the likely meiotic products.
- In experienced hands, the accuracy of PGD is high and the risk of an affected pregnancy following PGD using a well-designed test is low.
- It is important to understand the limitations of FISH testing and carefully counsel patients regarding the relatively low pregnancy rates associated with PGD for chromosome translocations.
- Emerging studies using PCR microsatellite analysis and microarray technology might offer potential advantages over the use of FISH in PGD for chromosome rearrangements.

Further Reading

Bint SM, Ogilvie CM, Flinter FA, Khalaf Y, Scriven PN. Meiotic segregation of Robertsonian translocations ascertained in cleavage-stage embryos – implications for preimplantation genetic diagnosis. Hum Reprod. 2011;26:1575–84.

Fiorentino F, Kokkali G, Biricik A, Stavrou D, Ismailoglu B, De Palma R, Arizzi L, Harton G, Sessa M, Pantos K. Polymerase chain reaction-based detection of chromosomal imbalances on embryos: the evolution of preimplantation genetic diagnosis for chromosomal translocations. Fertil Steril. 2010;94:2001–11.

Fiorentino F, Spizzichino L, Bono S, Biricik A, Kokkali G, Rienzi L, Ubaldi FM, Iammarrone E, Gordon A, Pantos K. PGD for reciprocal and Robertsonian translocations using array comparative genomic hybridization. Hum Reprod. 2011;26:1925–35.

Franssen MT, Korevaar JC, van der Veen F, Leschot NJ, Bossuyt PM, Goddijn M. Reproductive outcome after chromosome analysis in couples with two or more miscarriages: index [corrected]-control study. BMJ. 2006;332:759–63.

Harper JC, Wilton L, Traeger-Synodinos J, Goossens V, Moutou C, Sengupta SB, Pehlivan Budak T, Renwick P, De Rycke M, Geraedts JP, Harton G. The ESHRE PGD Consortium: 10 years of data collection. Hum Reprod Update. 2012;18(3):234–47.

Harton GL, Harper JC, Coonen E, Pehlivan T, Vesela K, Wilton L, European Society for Human Reproduction and Embryology (ESHRE) PGD Consortium. ESHRE PGD consortium best practice guidelines for fluorescence in situ hybridization-based PGD. Hum Reprod. 2011;26:25–32.

Mackie Ogilvie C, Scriven PN. Preimplantation genetic diagnosis for chromosome rearrangements. In: Harper JC, editor. Preimplantation genetic diagnosis. 2nd ed. Cambridge: Cambridge University Press; 2009. p. 194–201.

Mackie Ogilvie C, Scriven PN. Preimplantation genetic diagnosis for sex-linked diseases and sex-selection for non-medical reasons. In: Harper JC, editor. Preimplantation genetic diagnosis. 2nd ed. Cambridge: Cambridge University Press; 2009. p. 230–5.

Scriven PN, Bossuyt PM. Diagnostic accuracy: theoretical models for preimplantation genetic testing of a single nucleus using the fluorescence in situ hybridization technique. Hum Reprod. 2010;25:2622–8.

Scriven PN, Ogilvie CM. Fluorescence in situ hybridization on single cells. (Sex determination and chromosome rearrangements). Methods Mol Med. 2007;132:19–30.

Scriven PN, Handyside AH, Ogilvie CM. Chromosome translocations: segregation modes and strategies for preimplantation genetic diagnosis. Prenat Diagn. 1998;18:1437–49.

Scriven PN, Kirby TL, Ogilvie CM. FISH for pre-implantation genetic diagnosis. J Vis Exp. 2011;(48):pii: 2570. doi:10.3791/2570.

Treff NR, Northrop LE, Kasabwala K, Su J, Levy B, Scott Jr RT. Single nucleotide polymorphism microarray-based concurrent screening of 24-chromosome aneuploidy and unbalanced translocations in preimplantation human embryos. Fertil Steril. 2011;95:1606–12.

Chapter 8
PGD Analysis of Embryos for Monogenic Disorders

Pamela Renwick and Gheona Altarescu

The term monogenic disorder describes inherited disease caused by a defect in a single gene and encompasses those inherited in an autosomal recessive pattern (e.g. cystic fibrosis), autosomal dominant (e.g. myotonic dystrophy) and sex-linked (e.g. Duchenne muscular dystrophy). Most PGD for monogenic disorders is undertaken for couples at risk of having an offspring with life-limiting childhood onset disorders, but there is also a growing number of late-onset disorders (e.g. Huntington disease) and those with incomplete penetrance for which PGD is considered (e.g. hereditary breast cancer susceptibility) (Table 8.1).

In order to offer a couple PGD, the causative gene and the underlying mutation are confirmed in the family to allow the design of a specific genetic test to identify embryos unaffected by the disease. A demand on PGD centres is to provide equity of access to the PGD service when couples

P. Renwick, FCRPath, PhD, MSc, BSc (✉)
Assisted Conception Unit and PGD Centre,
Guy's and St. Thomas' Hospital NHS Foundation Trust,
11th Floor Tower Wing, Guy's Hospital, Great Maze Pond,
London SE1 9RT, UK
e-mail: pamela.renwick@gstt.nhs.uk

G. Altarescu, MD
Preimplantation Genetic Unit, Shaare Zedek Medical Center,
Medical Genetics Institute, Bayth Str. 12, Jerusalem 91031, Israel
e-mail: gheona@szmc.org.il

T. El-Toukhy, P. Braude (eds.), *Preimplantation Genetic
Diagnosis in Clinical Practice*, DOI 10.1007/978-1-4471-2948-6_8,
© Springer-Verlag London 2014

TABLE 8.1 Example monogenic diseases for which PGD can be undertaken, listed by inheritance mode. The disease, OMIM number and gene are given for reference

Autosomal recessive

Beta thalassaemia, 613985; HBB

Cystic fibrosis, 219700; CFTR

Epidermolysis bullosa-Herlitz junctional, 226700; LAMB3

Polycystic kidney disease, 263200; PKHD1

Sickle-cell anaemia, 603903; HBB

Spinal muscular atrophy, 253300; SMN1

Tay–Sachs, 272899; HEXA

Autosomal dominant

Breast cancer, 604370; BRCA1

Familial adenomatous polyposis, 175100; APC

Huntington disease, 143100; HTT

Marfan syndrome, 154700; FBN1

Myotonic dystrophy, 160900; DMPK

Neurofibromatosis 1, 162200; NF1

von Hippel–Lindau, 193300; VHL

X-linked

Adrenoleukodystrophy, 300100; ABCD1

Alport syndrome, 301050, COL5A1

Charcot–Marie–Tooth disease, 302800; Cx32

Duchenne muscular dystrophy, 310200, DMD

Fragile X syndrome, 300624; FMR1

Haemophilia A, 306700, F8

Hydrocephalus, 307000; L1CAM

Wiskott–Aldrich syndrome, 301000; WAS

present requesting PGD for rare genetic disorders which require new test design. Once a test is available, an initial feasibility study is undertaken to confirm that PGD can be offered to a couple before embarking on a PGD cycle.

Molecular Approaches

Monogenic diseases are tested using DNA amplification-based methodologies. In particular, polymerase chain reaction (PCR)-based assays are used to enrich selected sequences of the genome for genetic analysis. The very small amount of DNA (picograms) available from a single cell requires technical innovation to develop and maintain a sufficiently precise PCR test; most standard protocols used in diagnostic DNA laboratories are designed to use many nanograms of DNA and will not work on such tiny amounts of starting material.

Single-cell PCR procedures are extremely vulnerable to contamination by extraneous DNA and to allele dropout (ADO; where one or both of the two alleles at any locus fails to amplify) and preferential amplification of one allele over another, which compromises the accuracy of a diagnoses (Fig. 8.1). Therefore, intracytoplasmic sperm injection (ICSI) is used for all PCR-PGD cases as the presence of supernumerary sperm buried in the zona pellucida after IVF may result in contamination of PCR with paternal DNA. Conversely, oocytes are stripped of maternal cumulus cells to prevent contamination with maternal DNA as this could obscure the actual results in an embryo and result in a misdiagnosis.

Direct Mutation Testing

Specific mutations can be directly tested to provide a genotype; molecular techniques such as fragment size analysis, restriction site analysis, mini-sequencing and amplification refractory mutation systems (ARMS) have been utilised. If there is a common disease mutation, such as p.Phe508del

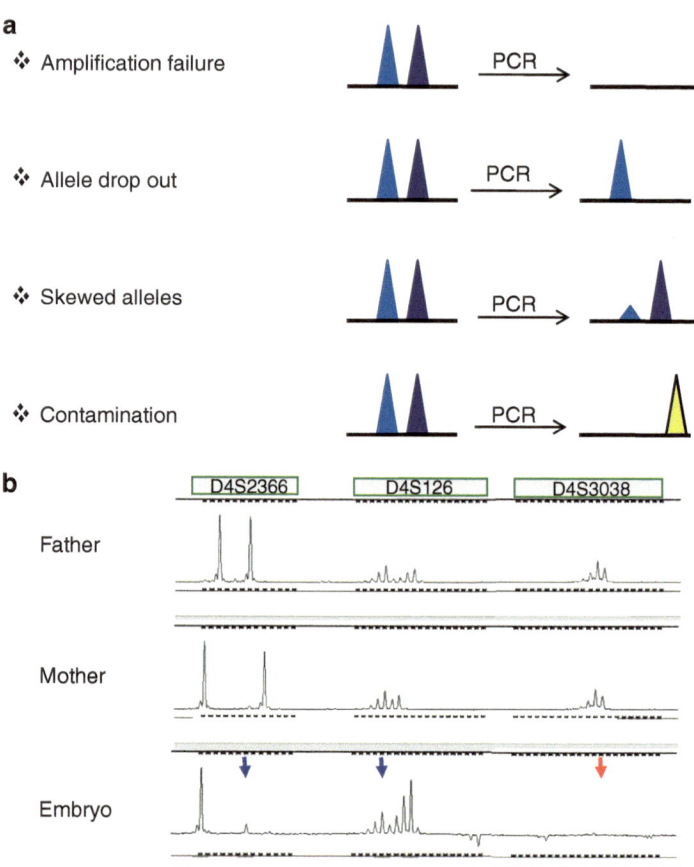

FIGURE. 8.1 (**a**) Problems encountered during single-cell PCR. (**b**) Electropherograms showing PCR of genomic DNA for father, mother and single cells for embryos E1 and E11 showing skewed amplification and a failed amplification for E11 at D4S3038

which accounts for 70 % of CF mutations in the North European population, then this test can be established at the single-cell level to offer to couples. In addition to the direct genotype test, several genetic markers linked to the gene should also be tested with the aim of reducing the misdiagnosis rate by controlling for ADO, monitoring for DNA contamination and confirming the mutation result by linkage analysis.

Indirect Testing by Linkage Analysis

Linkage analysis should be used wherever possible to back up the results of a direct mutation test offered in PGD. For disorders with heterogeneous mutations (e.g. over 1,000 different CF mutations are identified), a sole linkage approach can be used; this is more efficient and cost-effective than setting up mutation-specific tests for individual families. The use of three or more polymorphic markers substantially reduces the error rate due to ADO (from as high as 27 % in blastomeres for single amplicons to almost 0 %).

Most linkage analysis is carried out by using PCR to amplify microsatellite markers which are polymorphic short tandem repeats (STRs) located very close to or within the gene of interest. The STR markers are located close together along the chromosome and are inherited together; termed a haplotype and can be considered a mini-DNA fingerprint (Fig. 8.2). Markers are identified in a couple for which the STR sizes are sufficiently different between the couple to be informative to be used to identify and track the chromosome region (known as a haplotype) carrying the mutated gene in the family and hence in pre-implantation embryos (Fig. 8.3). However, there is a limit to the number of markers that can be simultaneously tested on a single cell without compromising the efficacy of the test, and only certain combinations of markers will work together at the single-cell level. A series of different linkage multiplexes therefore has to be available in order that the right combination can be offered to each couple, depending on which markers are informative.

In the case of sex-linked disorders for which the causative gene and mutation have been identified, testing for the disease status is often carried out in conjunction with looking at Y-chromosome markers for sex determination as only affected males are to be excluded. DNA-based approaches are preferred

Principle of haplotyping:
i) design primers for microsatellite markers either side of gene of interest
ii) amplify (from both chromosomes) by PCR
iii) separate products using capillary electrophoresis to give either:
2 products of different sizes, or
1 product (both alleles have same repeat length)

1) Genotype both partners and informative family member (eg affected child):

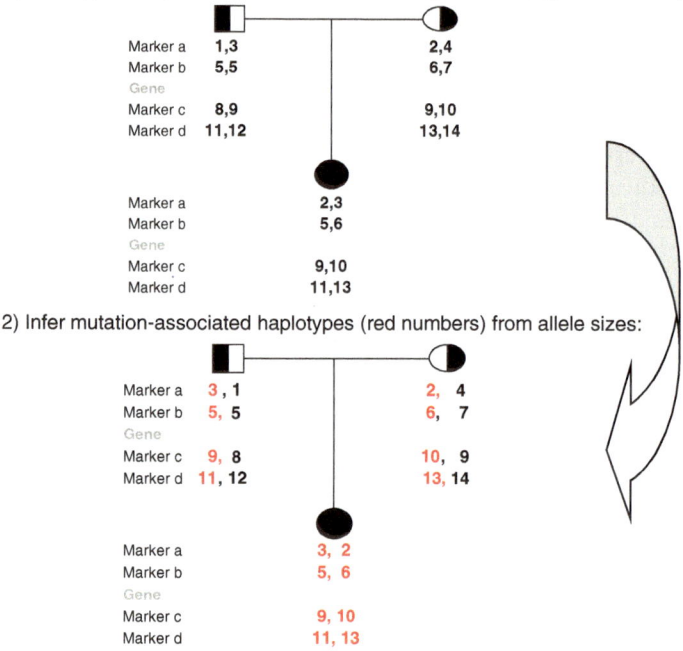

2) Infer mutation-associated haplotypes (red numbers) from allele sizes:

FIGURE. 8.2 Principle of haplotyping

over the use of FISH techniques, which can only identify and select female embryos for sex-linked recessive disease, resulting in the discarding all male embryos, 50 % of which are likely to be unaffected (Fig. 8.4). This practice not only raises ethical problems but also reduces the chances of pregnancy by depleting the number of embryos suitable for transfer.

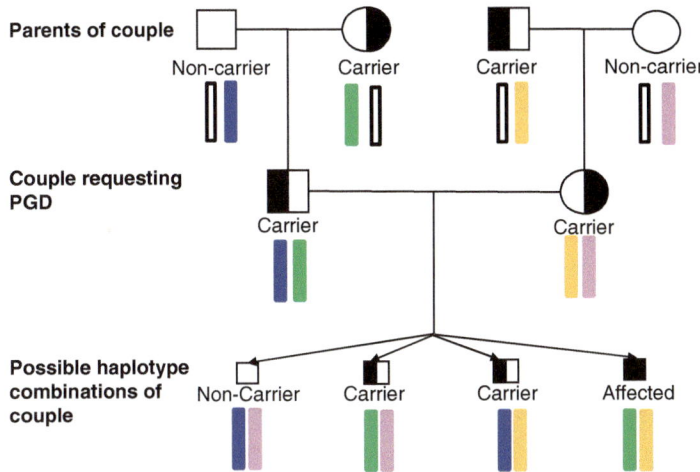

FIGURE. 8.3 Gene tracking in families using haplotyping and predicting the genetic status of future offspring for an autosomal recessive genetic disorder. The carrier/non-carrier status of family members needs to be known to assign phase to alleles to construct haplotypes (depicted as coloured bars). 1 in 4 offspring will be affected, 1 in 4 offspring will be unaffected non-carriers and 2 in 4 offspring will be unaffected carriers

Whole Genome Amplification

Whole genome amplification (WGA) overcomes the difficulties of testing single cells. There are several WGA methods but multiple displacement amplification (MDA) has been most widely used to date in PGD for monogenic disease due to its good coverage of the genome. Prior amplification by MDA of a single blastomere gives micrograms of DNA, which allows testing using standard DNA-based PCR protocols and the introduction of semiautomated sample handling. Other promising technologies are now emerging such as Omniplex.

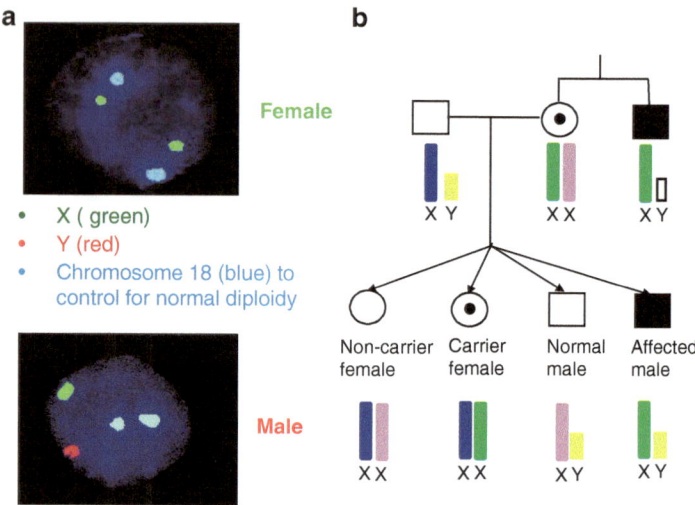

FIGURE. 8.4 Techniques used for X-linked disease. (**a**) FISH for sex determination of embryos; all males discarded even though half will be unaffected. (**b**) PGH for haplotyping and sex determination. Haplotypes created testing family members with known disease status (affected brother); PGH identifies carrier females and non-carrier females along with normal males; just affected male embryos are avoided

Preimplantation Genetic Haplotyping

PCR on MDA products shows ADO rates of approximately 20 %, which is unacceptably high to rely on direct mutation testing only, due to the likelihood of exclusion of embryos from transfer following inconclusive results. However, the problem of MDA-associated ADO can be overcome by indirect testing using multiple markers from within and around a disease gene to create haplotypes. Testing with a redundancy of markers means that even with high ADO, sufficient markers will amplify to allow haplotypes to be inferred. This approach has been termed preimplantation genetic haplotyping (PGH) and has been developed and applied clinically at Guy's PGD Centre since 2006 (Fig. 8.5; Table 8.2). Other

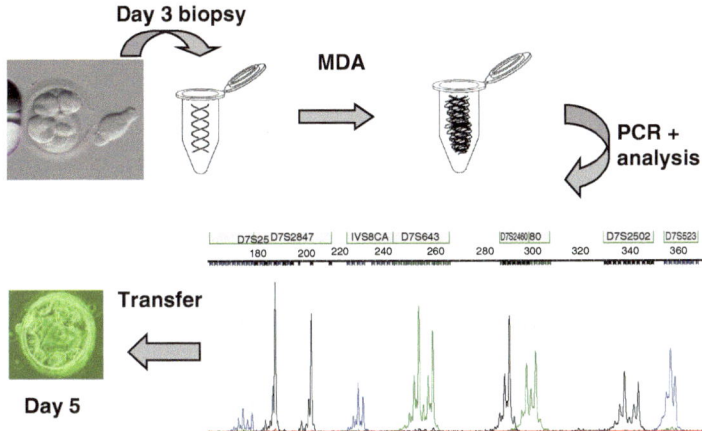

FIGURE. 8.5 Timeline for PGH involving a whole genome amplification step of MDA followed by PCR for haplotype analysis of embryos

groups have now introduced whole genome amplification and indirect haplotyping into their PGD programmes. The amount of amplified DNA available after MDA makes it possible to test for more than one monogenic disorder; PGH has been performed for couples where both are carriers of cystic fibrosis and in addition one partner is also a carrier of a second disease, such as haemophilia A, myotonic dystrophy or Wiskott–Aldrich syndrome (Fig. 8.6).

In addition, PGD tests using WGA utilise straightforward DNA-based tests which allow equitable access, as even couples with rare diseases can be offered PGD within a reasonable time frame. At Guy's, a tagged PCR approach is employed to fluorescently label DNA fragments for analysis, and the efficiency of test development and application means that cost savings can be passed on to patients and funding bodies.

Reliability and Limitations of Testing

PGD protocols must yield highly accurate results in a short period of time so that embryos can be transferred within the

TABLE 8.2 Outcomes of PGH cycles for autosomal recessive disease (AR;1 in 4 risk of an affected pregnancy), autosomal dominant (AD;1 in 2 risk) and X-linked recessive (XL;1 in 4 risk of an affected male). The mean age of the female partner was 33.4 years (range 21–41 years), for each genetic risk category, the following is given: the number of couples, tested biopsy cycles undertaken, cycles that reached embryo transfer (ET), cycles achieving a positive hCG pregnancy test, subsequent fetal heart beat positive clinical pregnancy (FHB+) and babies born. The clinical pregnancy rate per cycle that reached ET and per biopsy cycle are listed for comparison

| | Risk of affected pregnancy: | | |
	AR; 1 in 4	AD; 1 in 2	XL; 1 in 4
Couples	50	51	40
Biopsy cycles	57	68	54
Cycles to embryo transfer	52 (91 %)	58 (85 %)	53 (98 %)
Pregnancy (hCG+)	32	31	33
Clinical pregnancy (FHB+)	23	24	21
CPR/biopsy cycle	40 %	35 %	39 %
CPR/ET	44 %	41 %	40 %
CPR/couple	46 %	47 %	53 %
Babies born	26	25	24

window of successful implantation. For haplotyping, when results are obtained at multiple markers flanking the gene, then the associated misdiagnosis rate is the chance a double recombination event, resulting in the 'low risk' haplotype now harbouring the disease (<<1 %). To date worldwide, 12 misdiagnoses have been reported for a total of 2,400 PCR-based PGD cycles. Most of these are likely to have been due to allele dropout or undetected contamination with extraneous DNA or PCR products. A dense marker haplotype approach like PGH circumvents these problems with its mini-DNA fingerprint and substantially reduces the risk of misdiagnosis as it monitors contamination and confirms sample identity.

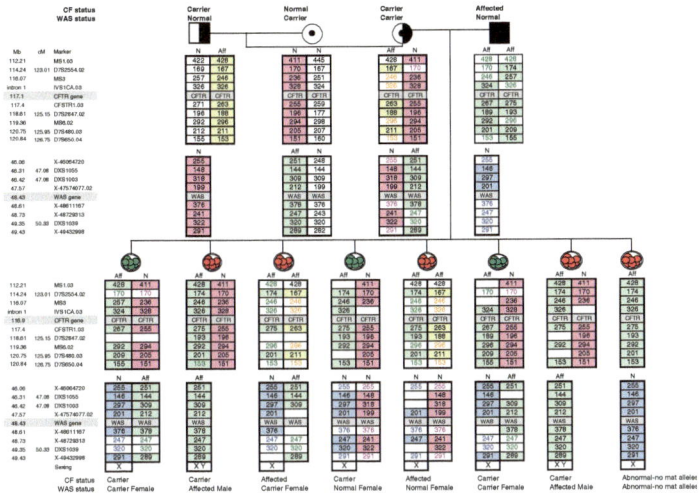

FIGURE. 8.6 Example results of PGH for a couple with a risk of having affected children with two inherited diseases of cystic fibrosis (autosomal recessive) and Wiskott–Aldrich syndrome (X-linked recessive). Thirteen embryos were biopsied (not all shown) and haplotyping for the CFTR and the WAS genes, along with sex determination undertaken. Four embryos were suitable for transfer; a single embryo was transferred resulting in a singleton delivery of a CF and WAS carrier female

It is expected to obtain a genetic diagnosis in approximately 90 % of embryos tested. The morphological quality of the embryo reflects the quality of the DNA in the biopsied cell for testing, and no, or doubtful, results are often obtained in embryos of low morphological quality with a low chance of implantation (Fig. 8.7).

Linkage/haplotype analysis depends upon the testing of markers within, or in close proximity to, the gene of interest to reduce errors caused by recombination. The ability to use linkage analysis depends on the availability of appropriate family samples to identify which chromosome carries the disease-causing gene (determination of phase). For various reasons, samples are not always available. Some couples are

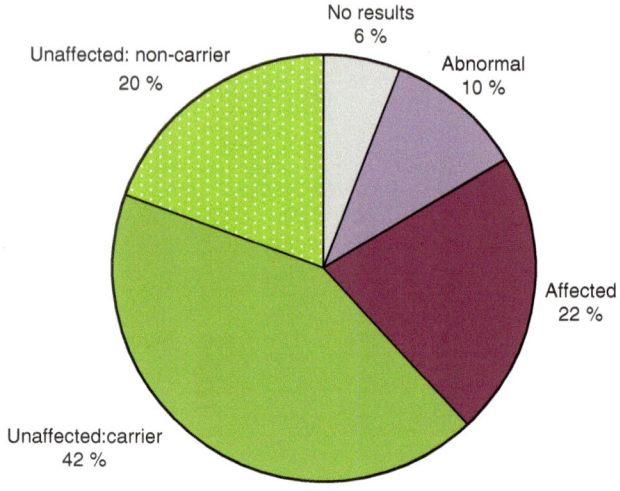

a   Autosomal recessive; 1 in 4 risk 448 embryos

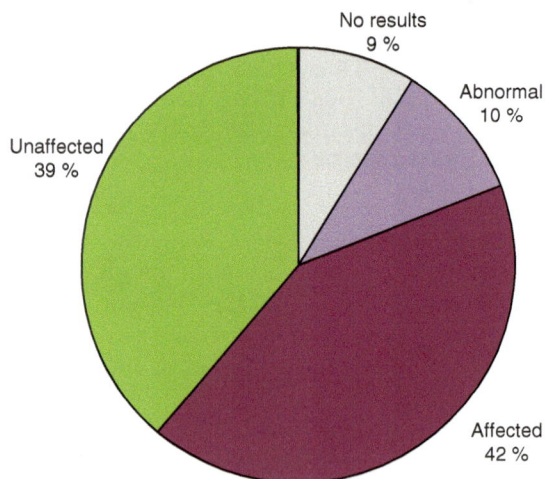

b   Autosomal dominant; 1 in 2 risk 469 embryos

FIGURE. 8.7 Embryo status categories obtained by PGH cycles for autosomal recessive (**a**) and for autosomal dominant disease (**b**). Embryos with possible aneuploidy for the chromosome tested (observed monosomy or trisomy) are scored as abnormal. Green depicts results that are genetically suitable for transfer (unaffected or carrier)

not willing to approach their families as they prefer not to reveal that they are considering PGD. Alternatively, they may not wish the familial genetic disease (such as Huntington disease) to be disclosed to the unaffected partner's family.

Sometimes the nature of the familial mutation may not be readily amenable to single-cell analysis, such as the case of triple-repeat diseases in which the expanded mutation cannot be amplified in single cells (such as CGG repeats in Fragile X or CTG repeats in myotonic dystrophy type 1). In these cases the PGD analysis is based solely on linkage analysis between affected and unaffected family members. As in all PGD cases, at least three informative markers surrounding the mutation should be included into the PGD analysis in order to ensure accuracy of the diagnosis and detect possible recombination events.

Special Considerations

Although molecular PGD can be theoretically performed for any genetic disorder with a known gene, there are several disorders where special considerations must be taken into account.

Facioscapulohumeral Muscular Dystrophy

Facioscapulohumeral muscular dystrophy (FSHD) (OMIM#158900) is the third most common hereditary muscle disease after Duchenne muscular dystrophy and myotonic dystrophy, with an estimated prevalence of 1 in 15,000. FSHD1A locus has been mapped at the 4q35.2 subtelomeric region, which contains a polymorphic microsatellite D4Z4 repeat consisting of 3.3-kb KpnI units varying in numbers between 11 and 150 copies. FSHD is commonly associated with the heterozygous contraction of 4q-D4Z4 arrays between 1 and 11 repeats. The molecular diagnosis is difficult, offered by only a few specialised laboratories, and requires large amounts of genomic DNA that are not applicable for single-cell analysis. An indirect method using linked polymorphic markers can be used, but the relatively high recombination risk could cause a higher rate of misdiagnosis compared with other monogenic disorders. Thus, special counselling should be given for patients with FSHD when performing PGD.

mtDNA

Mitochondrial disorders are often fatal multisystem diseases. A crucial characteristic of most pathogenic mtDNA mutations is heteroplasmy, the coexistence of normal and mutated mtDNA, requiring a threshold of mutated mtDNA to be exceeded before clinical symptoms occur. Expression thresholds and genotype–phenotype correlations have been evaluated for some of the common mtDNA mutations, but in most cases it is not possible to accurately predict the clinical manifestations based on the mutation load. For most (private) mtDNA point mutations, the information to judge this is not even available. The inability to predict the clinical expression very much limits the scope for both PGD and prenatal diagnosis to prevent the transmission of mtDNA disorders. Therefore, PGD of heteroplasmic mtDNA mutations should be based on adequate counselling and careful consideration of the uncertainties due to heteroplasmic levels of mutations in oocytes.

PGD for De Novo Mutations and Germline Mosaicism

Rarely, monogenic disease can appear 'de novo' in an individual, and the causative mutation is not present in the parents. In these instances there is a residual risk of a parent being a germline mosaic carrier of the mutation with the associated risk of recurrence of the genetic disorder with a further affected child. If the de novo-affected individual is requesting PGD, his or her gametes need to be tested for the mutation and linked markers so as to construct and assign normal and mutant haplotypes.

Germline mosaicism complicates allele assignment when constructing haplotypes for PGD since not all cells harbour the mutation. Single sperm or polar bodies (PB) may be used to define the origin of the high-risk haplotype (paternal or maternal origin) for accurate PGD analysis. To identify the high-risk allele in female mosaics, the haplotype analysis must be done with polar body PGD analysis. In cases in which paternal origin is suspected (based on haplotype analysis of parents and affected child), single-sperm analysis can confirm the presence of the mutation in a percentage of sperm. For males with de novo mutations, analysis of the haploid content of single sperm before the couple start the PGD cycle allows the setting of allelic phase and establishment of linked haplotypes. This method is also applicable in establishing linked haplotypes of any paternal mutation when linkage cannot be performed due to absence of other affected relatives.

Use of Polar Body Analysis

Polar bodies contain a chromosomal complement of the oocyte, so molecular analysis of PBs allows conclusions to be drawn on the genetic status of a specific oocyte. Polar body-based PGD has been shown to be an effective method for autosomal and X-linked dominant diseases, where the women is affected, and is possible in recessive disorders as well. This method has several advantages:

1. It allows embryo analysis without the removal of any embryonic cells.
2. If the PB analysis is inconclusive, a repeat analysis using a single blastomere can be performed at the 6–8 cell stage.
3. ADO rates have been observed to be significantly less in polar bodies than in blastomeres.
4. Informative markers are easier to identify since only the maternal alleles are present.

PB analysis requires oocyte retrieval so a protocol for real-time haplotype analysis during the PGD cycle using polar bodies 1 and 2 has to be performed. PB1, the result of meiosis I, can be either homozygous (no crossovers between the two alleles) or heterozygous (when crossing over occurs). Homozygous PB1s contain either the normal or mutant allele, while the other allele remains in the oocyte. PB2 is the result of meiosis II (post-fertilisation) and contains only one allele. Homozygote PB1s which show only one allele must be viewed as suspect for ADO, and therefore embryo transfer based on mutation detection alone can still lead to misdiagnosis. Mutation and linked markers can be tested, although sufficient oocytes need to be analysed to link the markers to the mutation and allow the transfer of unaffected embryos.

Key Points
- Direct mutation analysis along with linked markers on DNA from single cells provides an acceptable PGD assay but requires a lot of initial and ongoing test optimisation.
- PGD tests using WGA allow testing with standard DNA-based tests; haplotyping has the advantage over the disease-specific tests being applicable to all couples known to have a mutation in the disease gene.
- PGD for sex-linked disorders is moving from FISH-based sex selection to PCR-based mutation or haplotype analysis.
- Developing PGD tests is now faster and more efficient, allowing more equity of access for couples with rare disorders.

Further Reading

Altarescu G, Eldar-Geva T, Varshower I, Brooks B, Haran EZ, Margalioth EJ, Levy-Lahad E, Renbaum PPI. Real-time reverse linkage using polar body analysis for preimplantation genetic diagnosis in female carriers of de novo mutations. Hum Reprod. 2009;24(12):3225–9.

Altarescu G, Beeri R, Eldar-Geva T, Varshaver I, Margalioth EJ, Levy-Lahad E, Renbaum P. PGD for germline mosaicism. Reprod Biomed Online. 2012;25(4):390–5.

Barat-Houari M, Nguyen K, Bernard R, Fernandez C, Vovan C, Bareil C, Khau Van Kien P, Thorel D, Tuffery-Giraud S, Vasseur F, Attarian S, Pouget J, Girardet A, Lévy N, Claustres M. New multiplex PCR-based protocol allowing indirect diagnosis of FSHD on single cells: can PGD be offered despite high risk of recombination? Eur J Hum Genet. 2010;18(5):533–8.

Fiorentino F, Magli MC, Podini D, Ferraretti AP, Nuccitelli A, Vitale N, Baldi M, Gianaroli L. The minisequencing method: an alternative strategy for preimplantation genetic diagnosis of single gene disorders. Mol Hum Reprod. 2003;9:399–410.

Goossens V, Traeger-Synodinos J, Coonen E, De Rycke M, Moutou C, Pehlivan T, Derks-Smeets IA, Harton G. ESHRE PGD consortium data collection XI: cycles from January to December 2008 with pregnancy follow-up to October 2009. Hum Reprod. 2012;27(7):1887–911.

Handyside AH, Robinson MD, Simpson RJ, Omar MB, Shaw MA, Grudzinskas JG, Rutherford A. Isothermal whole genome amplification from single and small numbers of cells: a new era for preimplantation genetic diagnosis of inherited disease. Mol Hum Reprod. 2004;10:767–72.

Handyside AH, Harton GL, Mariani B, Thornhill AR, Affara N, Shaw MA, Griffin DK. Karyomapping: a universal method for genome wide analysis of genetic disease based on mapping crossovers between parental haplotypes. J Med Genet. 2010;47(10):651–8.

Harper JC, Wilton L, Traeger-Synodinos J, Goossens V, Moutou C, SenGupta SB, Pehlivan Budak T, Renwick P, De Rycke M, Geraedts JP, Harton G. The ESHRE PGD consortium: 10 years of data collection. Hum Reprod Update. 2012;18(3):234–47.

Harton GL, De Rycke M, Fiorentino F, Moutou C, SenGupta S, Traeger-Synodinos J, Harper JC, European Society for Human Reproduction and Embryology (ESHRE). PGD consortium. ESHRE PGD consortium best practice guidelines for amplification-based PGD. Hum Reprod. 2010;26(1):33–40.

Hellebrekers DMEI, Wolfe R, Hendrick ATM, de Coo IFM, de Die CE, Geraedts JPM, Chinnery PF, Smeets HJM. PGD and heteroplasmic mitochondrial DNA point mutations: a systematic review estimating the chance of healthy offspring. Hum Reprod Update. 2012;18(4): 341–9.

Poulton J, Chiaratti MR, Meirelles FV, Kennedy S, Wells D, Holt IJ. Transmission of mitochondrial DNA diseases and ways to prevent them. PLoS Genet. 2010;6(8):pii: e1001066.

Rechitsky S, Pomerantseva E, Pakhalchuk T, Pauling D, Verlinsky O, Kuliev A. First systematic experience of preimplantation genetic diagnosis for de-novo mutations. Reprod Biomed Online. 2011;22(4):350–61. Epub 2011 Jan 20.

Renwick P, Ogilvie CM. Preimplantation genetic diagnosis for monogenic diseases: overview and emerging issues. Expert Rev Mol Diagn. 2007;7:33–43.

Renwick PJ, Trussler J, Ostad-Saffari E, Fassihi H, Black C, Braude P, Ogilvie CM, Abbs S. Proof of principle and first cases using preimplantation genetic haplotyping-a paradigm shift for embryo diagnosis. Reprod Biomed Online. 2006;13:110–9.

Renwick P, Trussler J, Lashwood A, Braude P, Ogilvie CM. Preimplantation genetic haplotyping: 127 diagnostic cycles demonstrating a robust, efficient alternative to direct mutation testing on single cells. Reprod Biomed Online. 2010;20(4):470–6.

Sermon K, De Rycke M. Single cell polymerase chain reaction for preimplantation genetic diagnosis: methods, strategies, and limitations. Methods Mol Med. 2007;132:31–42.

Wilton L, Thornhill A, Traeger-Synodinos J, Sermon KD, Harper JC. The causes of misdiagnosis and adverse outcomes in PGD. Hum Reprod. 2009;24(5):1221–8.

Chapter 9
Managing the PGD Cycle

Yacoub Khalaf and Jan Grace

PGD is a multidisciplinary process involving not only clinical and paramedical professionals members but administrative team members who have a crucial role to play in ensuring a smooth process and that patients are satisfied with the way that their cycle has been handled. Each member of the team has their specific role but may not see through the entire process, each playing their part when needed. Nevertheless they each should be aware of the sequence and stages involved in the PGD cycle in order to be able to provide correct helpful information to the patient when requested. Efficiency of the process can be facilitated by the use of checklists to ensure that crucial details are not omitted at each stage.

Y. Khalaf, MBBCh, MSc, MD, FRCOG, MFFP (✉)
J. Grace, BSc, MBBS, MRCOG
Assisted Conception Unit, Guy's and St. Thomas Hospital NHS Foundation Trust, 11th Floor, Tower Wing, Great Maze Pond, London, SE1 9RT, UK
e-mail: yakoub.khalaf@kcl.ac.uk; jan.grace@gstt.nhs.uk

T. El-Toukhy, P. Braude (eds.), *Preimplantation Genetic Diagnosis in Clinical Practice*, DOI 10.1007/978-1-4471-2948-6_9,
© Springer-Verlag London 2014

A Typical PGD Pathway

Processing the Request

Couples with a history of a genetic condition, or if a recent discovery following the birth of an affected child, will usually be referred to a specialist genetic centre. However this may not be the case in recurrent miscarriage involving a chromosome rearrangement identified as part of gynaecological or fertility investigations where a direct referral from the gynaecologist or general practitioner may be received.

Ideally the couple will be assessed by a local geneticist who already may be familiar with the couple and their genetic condition through looking after them and/or their affected child (ren), or as a new referral in order to discuss PGD in principle among other reproductive options available.

Part of the geneticists' role should ensure that the couples seeking PGD have a full assessment of their genetic condition, its health implications including a medical assessment if needed and alternative therapeutic options if any. This is in order to satisfy themselves that the particular genetic condition poses a significant risk of serious physical/or mental disability to warrant PGD and that PGD is feasible and appropriate.

Couples expressing interest in further exploring PGD should be referred to the PGD programme by the geneticist.

Counselling Appointment

The PGD counsellor reviews the referral ensuring key points are available in order for a specialist counselling appointment to be given (Checklist 1).

Checklist 1

- Genetic condition reviewed including ascertainment of the diagnosis, its mode of inheritance and the advisability of PGD and availability of a suitable PGD test

- Explanation of what's involved in PGD including the diagnostic workup, preparation of a specific test to detect the affected gene/chromosome in their embryos and the general process of IVF, including its potential risks and complications, in order to produce embryos
- The decision about the number and genetic status of embryos to transfer
- Alternative reproductive options
- Patients who wish to proceed with the PGD option are asked to provide blood samples. Blood samples may be necessary from their parents or from any affected sibling or parent in order to prepare the appropriate diagnostic workup
- Licensing application is made to the HFEA for those conditions that are not already licensed in the UK

Diagnostic Workup Period

This part of the process may be variable depending whether a test is already available or whether a specific test for the couple needs to be designed. Workup times for new tests may be prolonged (up to 6 months), but with increasing sophistication and mechanisation of testing, most tests can be available within a shorter period (6 weeks).

If a suitable test is available or has been designed, the patient is invited to attend the assisted conception unit for a consultation with one of the IVF specialists.

Assisted Conception Specialist Appointment

Part of the assisted conception specialists' role is to ensure that the patient is medically suitable for PGD and clear about what is involved in the process including all the different steps, chances of a healthy live birth, risks and complications (and measures to minimise them) and provide the reproductive care required for PGD (Checklist 2). They are also expected to consider the welfare of any child resulting from PGD. Assisted conception specialists are expected to involve medical practitioners from other disciplines whenever appropriate (refer to Chap. 5).

Checklist 2

- A full medical history is taken from both partners.
- Clinical examination of female partners (and male partners when required).
- A baseline transvaginal ultrasound scan is performed to assess the pelvis for any abnormality that could interfere with success of treatment. Any issues that are picked up would be dealt with appropriately after counselling the patient about the implications of abnormal results and proposed treatment (see Chap. 5).
- The male partner has a semen analysis or result of any previous analysis discussed. A surgical sperm retrieval procedure is planned for azoospermic men.
- For the female partner a test of ovarian reserve (Chap. 5) is arranged.
- The couple are screened for HIV, Hepatitis B and Hepatitis C as required by HFEA. Rubella immunity is established in the female. Any other tests such as haemoglobinopathy and additional genetic tests, e.g. Tay-Sachs and CF screen arranged if applicable.
- The treatment cycle is explained including the potential risks and side effects. The relevant consent forms are completed for treatment procedures including oocyte retrieval, fertilisation, embryos biopsy, transfer, cryo-storage and research options. The results of the genetic diagnostic workup and the small risk of misdiagnosis are discussed. We also discuss our single-embryo transfer policy and discuss the risks of multiple pregnancy.
- Provided no extra information is required or treatment needed, the couple should be ready to start treatment.

The Treatment Process (Fig. 9.1)

Typically patients will have their menstrual cycle programmed using the oral contraceptive pill (OCP) in order to help with scheduling the timing of their treatment. Some

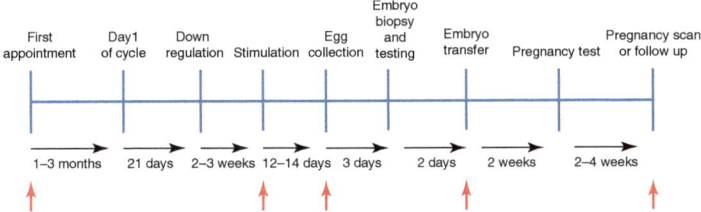

FIGURE 9.1 Timeline of a PGD treatment cycle

women may already be using the OCP to avoid an affected pregnancy. The day of their withdrawal bleed can be manipulated so that the throughput of patients can be moderated to accommodate as many patients as is safe and to fit in with the available capacity of the PGD programme.

Patients are asked to stop the OCP on a defined day. A few days later, when they start their withdrawal (menstrual) bleed, they are usually commenced on medication to suppress their endogenous hormonal cycle (using nasal spray or injections to suppress the pituitary gland). This pituitary suppression (downregulation) agent usually takes 2 weeks to achieve the desired effect of ovarian quiescence.

When downregulation is achieved, as demonstrated on transvaginal ultrasound by the appearances of inactive ovaries and a thin endometrium, ovarian stimulation using gonadotropins is commenced. Pituitary suppression by nasal spray or injection is continued simultaneously in order to prevent the possibility of a natural LH surge that would induce premature ovulation. This regime is continued for 2 weeks during which time FSH injections are self-administered daily to stimulate the development of egg-containing follicles in the ovary. Appropriate monitoring of response to ovarian stimulation is performed usually using ultrasound scans. Where there is an increased risk of OHSS, monitoring of ovarian response to stimulation is begun earlier (day 5 or 6 of stimulation) and serial serum estradiol blood tests arranged so that the dose of gonadotropins may be adjusted or its administration withheld.

After about 2 weeks, when the ovaries contain follicles deemed to be of a size (around 18 mm) and number most likely to contain an adequate number of mature eggs, oocyte pick up is scheduled.

Timings are given for precise administration of hCG or LH. The hCG injection is given around 34–36 h before the time scheduled for egg collection.

When eggs are collected they are fertilised with partner/husband's sperm. In PGD for single-gene disorders, ICSI is usually used routinely, whereas for sexing and chromosomal rearrangement, ICSI is used only when the sperm is judged inadequate for conventional IVF.

For cleavage-stage biopsy, the fertilised eggs are incubated for 3 days when they usually contain six to eight cells. Blastocyst stage biopsy when many more cells are available requires that the embryos be kept in culture for between 5 and 6 days.

Test results are available the following day following biopsy. The embryologist or genetic counsellor will ring the patient with the results and plan for embryo transfer.

Unaffected embryos are transferred on day 5 of development. Patients are strongly advised to have a single blastocyst transferred at a time in order to avoid multiple pregnancy with its well-documented risks and complications. Any additional tested embryos that are suitable for transfer are frozen and stored for future use by the couple. Embryos that are unsuitable for transfer are either donated for research/training or discarded according the couple's wishes and their informed consent.

Patients are informed as to what should happen in the days after the embryo transfer. Progesterone for luteal support is continued and a urine pregnancy test is performed 10–11 days after embryo transfer.

Patients who have a positive pregnancy test are offered a pregnancy scan 2–3 weeks after the positive test. Patients whose pregnancy test is negative are offered a follow-up appointment to discuss the details of their cycle and advise whether further attempts are recommended. Some couple may find supportive counselling helpful under these circumstances.

Once viability of a pregnancy is established, patients are referred to their local hospital for antenatal care. They are asked to provide the PGD centre with information about the outcome of their pregnancy, and cord blood samples for diagnostic confirmation were applicable.

Satellite PGD

As PGD is a highly specialised tertiary service, patients may be referred from a wide geographical area to the PGD centre. Devolving part of the pathway to be conducted locally makes patients' treatment pathway easier and reduces the need for long-distance travel without compromising the overall quality of the process.

The satellite centre takes care of initial genetic assessment and PGD counselling in addition to the reproductive care required for preparing the patient for the oocyte retrieval.

The treatment pathway is coordinated with the PGD centre, and the information collected from monitoring ovarian stimulation is shared with the PGD centre in a timely manner so that PGD cycle can be managed in accordance with the centre's scheduling scheme.

Provision of adequate information, clear communication from different members of the highly specialised PGD team, managing expectations and emotional support throughout the PGD cycle are essential to achieving a satisfactory patient experience. Patients should be made aware of the time required for the preparatory steps before their treatment can be initiated. Care should be taken to avoid the two most serious complications of the IVF process (OHSS and multiple pregnancy) as the process should not substitute reducing the risk posed to the pregnancy by the genetic disorder by risks posed the iatrogenic complication of the process.

An Alternative Approach to the PGD Cycle: Dislocation

Following egg collection and fertilisation, embryos are incubated in the embryology laboratory for 5–6 days. Embryos that reach the blastocyst stage are biopsied and then frozen using vitrification (flash freezing) and stored.

The biopsy obtained from each embryo is now available for testing without the pressure of an immediate result. Testing for the relevant genetic/chromosomal abnormality can be scheduled within 2 weeks of biopsy.

Patients are informed of their results as soon as they are available and confirmed.

An appointment can be made immediately to discuss any adverse results where there are no embryos for transfer. Those who have embryos that are deemed suitable for transfer will be offered a date to have one of their frozen embryos thawed and replaced into the uterus in a medicated or natural menstrual cycle.

Advantages of this approach:

- Improved safety and effectiveness of ovarian stimulation as the risk of OHSS can be significantly reduced through the use of an alternative ovarian stimulation protocol.
- Rapid access to treatment as it would enable couple to embark on assisted conception treatment as soon as their diagnostic workup is complete without having to wait until a slot for biopsy and testing becomes available.
- The duration of the PGD cycle would be markedly reduced; a shorter stimulation regime can be used. These can be started from day 1 of the menstrual cycle or withdrawal bleed and do not require the long period of downregulation. Embryos would be ready for biopsy in 3 weeks instead of 7–8 weeks in the other approach.
- Improved efficiency of embryo testing; testing can be conducted in batches allowing weekday working for staff and coordinating resources and consumables. More staff can

be allocated working together which improves safety of checking, sharing and discussing results.
- Potential improved overall outcome of treatment as there some evidence to suggest that babies resulting from frozen-thawed embryo transfer cycles have higher birth weight and are at lower risk of being born prematurely.

Key Points
- PGD is a multidisciplinary process involving clinical, paramedical, laboratory, and nursing professionals, and an administrative team who have a crucial role to play in ensuring a smooth process and that patients are satisfied with the way that their cycle has been handled.
- Each member of the team has their specific role but may not see through the entire process, each playing their part when needed.
- Nevertheless all should be aware of the sequence and stages involved in the PGD cycle in order to be able to provide correct helpful information to the patient when requested.
- The pathway involves in sequence, administrative processing of the request, review by geneticist or genetic counsellor, and a diagnostic workup period by the laboratory before the reproductive specialist can individualise a treatment plan for the couple.
- A typical cycle from first genetic appointment to egg collection may take anywhere from 12 to 20 weeks, followed by another week for biopsy testing and embryo transfer, and possible cryopreservation. Hence expectations of immediate results must be managed sympathetically.

Chapter 10
Training and Accreditation in PGD

Frances Flinter, Caroline Mackie Ogilvie, Virginia N. Bolton, Alison Lashwood, and Tarek El-Toukhy

F. Flinter, MD, FRCP, FRCPCH, MB, BS, DCH (✉)
A. Lashwood, MSc, RGN, RSCN, DIPHV
Clinical Genetics Department, Guy's and St. Thomas' Hospital
NHS Foundation Trust, 7th Floor Borough Wing, Guy's Hospital,
Great Maze Pond, London SE1 9RT, UK
e-mail: frances.flinter@gstt.nhs.uk;
alison.lashwood@gstt.nhs.uk

C.M. Ogilvie, BSc, DPhil
Cytogenetics Department, Guy's and St. Thomas' Hospital NHS
Foundation Trust, 5th Floor, Tower Wing, Guy's Hospital,
Great Maze Pond, London SE1 9RT, UK
e-mail: caroline.ogilvie@genetics.kcl.ac.uk

V.N. Bolton, MA, PhD
T. El-Toukhy, MBBCh, MSc, MD, MRCOG
Assisted Conception Unit, Guy's and St. Thomas' Hospital NHS
Foundation Trust, 11th Floor, Tower Wing, Guy's Hospital,
Great Maze Pond, London SE1 9RT, UK
e-mail: virginia.bolton@gstt.nhs.uk;
tarek.el-toukhy@gstt.nhs.uk

T. El-Toukhy, P. Braude (eds.), *Preimplantation Genetic Diagnosis in Clinical Practice*, DOI 10.1007/978-1-4471-2948-6_10, © Springer-Verlag London 2014

PGD is a complex process that requires a large team with diverse but overlapping skill sets. For PGD to be safe and competently practised, each area requires high standards of clinical and laboratory practice. In the UK and throughout the EU, accreditation and training systems have been set in place to ensure quality and suitable training.

Clinical Genetics

Clinical genetics is the specialty concerned with the diagnosis of inherited disorders and birth defects, the estimation of genetic risk and genetic counselling of family members. Clinical geneticists work in multidisciplinary regional genetics centres in close collaboration with genetic counsellors, laboratory scientists and academic colleagues and play a central role in providing high-quality care for couples seeking PGD. They also work with colleagues across numerous medical specialties, professionals working in other areas such as social services and patient-support groups.

Clinical geneticists need a wide range of clinical skills as genetic disorders can affect people of all ages and involve all body systems. Communication skills are particularly important in explaining complex concepts and genetic test results in ways that enable people to make informed decisions. Clinical geneticists provide advice for other professionals and support the application of genetic and genomic technologies across the wider medical community.

Training Pathway

Specialty training in clinical genetics in the UK consists of core and higher specialty training. Core training may be completed through either core medical training, an acute care common stem programme, or level one paediatrics. By the end of this period, trainees acquire membership of the Royal College of Physicians (MRCP) or Paediatrics and Child Health (MRCPCH). The clinical genetics training then follows, leading to a certificate of completed training after a minimum of 72 months. The trainee is required to pass an exit certificate examination in clinical genetics. Trainees usually achieve competence in 6 years of the specialty training programme: 2 years core training, followed by 4 years clinical genetics training. Candidates may already have a BSc in genetics or an MSc in clinical genetics, and many undertake a significant period of research, leading to the award of a higher degree.

Key Skills and Attitudes

Trainees in clinical genetics learn to establish a genetic diagnosis by taking a family history, performing a physical examination and considering appropriate investigations, before providing advice and support for patients, and also their relatives, if indicated. During the course of their training, they must demonstrate that they have the knowledge, skills and attitudes required to manage time and problems effectively. It is essential that they understand and follow established principles, guidance and laws regarding medical ethics and confidentiality appropriately. This is particularly important when dealing with information that is relevant to several different members of a family, all of whom may be affected by, or at risk of, the same condition. Trainees must also become proficient in a small number of procedures, such as taking blood samples and skin biopsies from adults and children including those with special needs, extracting hair roots and taking appropriate photographs. Trainees also spend a period of time in the laboratory in order to acquire the skills and knowledge required to request and interpret specialised genetic laboratory tests within a clinical setting.

Subspecialties: A number of specific subspecialties are developing within the clinical genetics framework, including neurogenetics, cancer genetics, paediatric genetics, dysmorphology, prenatal diagnosis and fetal dysmorphology, and cardiac genetics.

Genetic Counsellors

In some PGD centres, the professionals offering genetic counselling will be either medically qualified clinical geneticists or genetic counsellors. Genetic counsellors will generally have higher education in either a nursing or science discipline, usually having undertaken a Masters-level degree in a related field.

Genetic counselling is a recognised accredited profession with differing regulatory frameworks across the world. Internationally, the availability, extent and quality of genetic counselling will vary. In the UK, unlike North America and Australia, a voluntary registration scheme based on the submission of a portfolio of evidence fulfilling required competencies has been in place since 2002. A UK scheme for national regulation is being developed through the Assured Voluntary Register (AVR) by the Health Professions Council.

Reproductive Medicine and PGD

PGD clinicians work as part of the wider multidisciplinary team, including but not restricted to clinical geneticists, genetic counsellors, molecular and cytogenetic scientists, specialist nurses, clinical embryologists and quality managers. They also interact regularly with healthcare professionals in other medical disciplines to ensure the provision of a comprehensive and high-standard service for couples seeking PGD treatment.

The Training Pathway

Training for gynaecologists involved in PGD treatment is undertaken as part of subspecialty training in reproductive medicine. Subspecialty training in reproductive medicine in the UK starts after completing at least 5 years of core training in general obstetrics and gynaecology and passing all the membership examinations of the Royal College of

Obstetricians and Gynaecologists (RCOG). This subspecialty training lasts for 2–3 years and has to be undertaken in an accredited tertiary level reproductive medicine centre. PGD training is undertaken in those centres which offer a PGD service.

By the end of subspecialty training, trainees will be expected to have completed one or more clinical research projects. Some trainees may electively undertake an out-of-programme fellowship programme for 1–2 years to gain further experience and complete a research project in reproductive medicine or PGD, which may lead to the award of a higher degree (MSc or MD). Candidates successful in completing all subspecialty training modules are awarded the Certificate of Completed Training (CCT) in Obstetrics and Gynaecology and Subspecialist Accreditation in Reproductive Medicine. Trainees usually achieve CCT and subspecialist accreditation after completing 7 or 8 years of a structured training programme, 5 years of core training and 2–3 years of subspecialist training. There is no exit certificate examination, but trainees are assessed by internal specialists, and through the RCOG and interview by external accredited subspecialists on a regular basis for competency achievement against agreed standards.

Skills and Attitudes

Clinical training in reproductive medicine and PGD requires a knowledge base and skill competence in assisted conception techniques, including pretreatment patient preparation, regimes of controlled ovarian stimulation, oocyte and sperm retrieval, embryo transfer and avoidance of related complications such as ovarian hyperstimulation syndrome and multiple pregnancy. Trainees in reproductive medicine complete structured training modules in accredited genetic centres, in which they develop an understanding of genetic inheritance and transmission of genetic disease, learn how to obtain a full genetic history and to counsel sensitively and appropriately couples at risk of transmitting genetic disease to their future child about their reproductive options. They also spend time in embryology and genetic laboratories acquiring knowledge about techniques of cell and embryo culture, biopsy and small sample DNA extraction and amplification and interpretation of test results. During their training, candidates must demonstrate full understanding of and compliance with the HFEA Code of Practice and specialist society (British Fertility Society) guidance with regard to assisted conception and PGD practice in the UK. They are also required to be familiar with the principles of medical and reproductive ethics, particularly those related to PGD and prenatal testing in general.

The Diagnostic Genetics Laboratory

Genetic testing for PGD should be carried out in accredited laboratories, using staff trained and registered appropriately for their roles.

Accreditation of genetic testing laboratories in the UK is achieved through the authorising body (currently Clinical Pathology Accreditation (UK) Ltd). Accredited status is awarded following a visit by external peer assessors who carry out an in-depth inspection against established standards that cover all aspects of the work including health and safety, all technical procedures, management of staff and premises and quality assurance. All laboratories must have a quality manager who has responsibility for ensuring that all the above areas comply with the standards on an ongoing basis and who prepares a quality manual that contains all documentation, including standard operating procedures (SOPs), a quality policy and departmental objectives. SOPs for all stages of all tests must be controlled to ensure that only the current version is in circulation and that they are subject to regular review. Accreditation recognises that the laboratory is competent to carry out all the procedures involved in PGD.

Laboratory competency is also monitored by external quality assessment (EQA) organised nationally or Europewide; annual rounds of assessment involve either the testing of material sent or submission of reports based on electronic images made available to the laboratory. Performance is assessed by accuracy of analysis and by the standard of the written reports submitted to quality assessors, and a mark is awarded to each laboratory. Laboratories with consistently low marks in these EQA schemes are labelled as "poor performers"; such laboratories should be required to improve their performance before further involvement in PGD.

The Training Pathway

Clinical scientists in the UK undergo a national training scheme following which they are eligible to be registered with the Health and Care Professions Council; this registration must be renewed biennially. Continual professional development and records of competency are required for registration, and evidence may be requested. Registration is also available for technical staff involved in PGD. In addition, structured training for the individual procedures required for PGD should be in place, with training logs and records of competencies for each procedure. Errors should be recorded, and regular performance review of each individual staff member should be carried out. All staff involved in PGD are required to be included on their clinic's HFEA licence and subject to the confidentiality restraints of the Human Fertilisation and Embryology Act.

The Assisted Conception Laboratory (Embryo Biopsy)

Fertilisation in vitro, embryo culture, biopsy for PGD and cryopreservation should be carried out in laboratories that are accredited, designated, authorised or licensed under national quality or safety laws. In the EU, laboratories undertaking procedures for assisted conception are required to have in place a quality management system that ensures traceability, not only of all gametes and embryos, but also of all materials or equipment that could have an impact on the quality and safety of the gametes and embryos, and must have been certified by an internationally recognised body. In the UK, these requirements are included among those that must be met before the issuing/renewal of a Treatment Licence by the Human Fertilisation and Embryology Authority (HFEA).

Training Pathway

Since 1993, formal training for clinical embryologists in the UK has been under the auspices of the Association of Clinical Embryologists (ACE). The postgraduate Certificate in Clinical Embryology has a minimum entry requirement of a degree in life sciences and requires a minimum of 2 years' full-time supervised training in the laboratories of a UK-based assisted conception unit, during and after which theoretical knowledge and competencies in practical skills are assessed. Within 3 years of commencing training, embryologists are eligible for assessment to be registered as clinical embryologists with the Health and Care Professions Council (HCPC). Continual professional development and records of competency are required for registration, and evidence may be requested.

Competency in embryo biopsy is not a requirement for registration with the HCPC, and centres are required by the HFEA to develop in-house processes for training and competency assessment in biopsy techniques, including criteria for evaluation and assessment of training progress of individual practitioners. Processes should be developed for each stage of development that is biopsied. Practitioners should maintain individual logs of procedures undertaken to enable regular performance review.

Key Points
- Structured training in the different professional disciplines is the cornerstone of providing a high standard of PGD practice.
- Although training requirements may vary across EU countries, regular review of the progress of the trainees will ensure that the required skills and competencies are achieved prior to final accreditation and/or state registration.
- Formal appraisal and regular performance reviews provide evidence that high standards of care are upheld.

Further Reading

http://www.embryologists.org.uk/Education/Education.

http://www.hpc-uk.org/assets/documents/10003850HPCpolicystatement-Voluntaryregistration.pdf.

http://www.jrcptb.org.uk/trainingandcert/ST3-SpR/Pages/Clinical-Genetics.aspx.

http://www.rcog.org.uk/curriculum-module/reproductive-medicine.

http://www.rcog.org.uk/files/rcog-corp/uploaded-files/ED-CCT-Regulations.pdf.

http://www.rcog.org.uk/files/rcog-corp/uploaded-files/ED-SUBSPEC-RM-Curriculum.pdf.

Skirton H, Barnes C, Guilbert P, Kershaw A, Kerzin-Storrar L, Patch C, Curtis G, Walford-Moore J. Recommendation for education and training of genetic nurses and counsellors in the UK. J Med Genet. 1998;35(5):410–2.

Chapter 11
PGD Data in the UK and Europe

Alan R. Thornhill and Paul N. Scriven

The purpose of data collection should be to provide accountability, assurance of safety and efficacy for patients and practitioners, promote best practice and suggest areas in which more improvements could be made. PGD outcomes have been collected in a variety of different ways by individual centres, professional bodies and regulatory agencies: it is a mandatory requirement of the HFEA to collect and make centre data publicly available, and data collection and publication has been one of the central objectives of the ESHRE PGD Consortium since its inception in 1997. This chapter explores the nature of these data, what is useful and what is not, and suggests possible future improvements. While acknowledging that many of the key points discussed are relevant to both PGS and PGD, this chapter will focus on data collected for PGD for single-gene disorders and chromosomal aberrations.

─────────

A.R. Thornhill, PhD (✉)
Assisted Conception Unit, Guy's Hospital, 11th Floor, Tower Wing, Guy's Hospital, Great Maze Pond, London SE1 9RT, UK
e-mail: alan.thornhill@gstt.nhs.uk

P.N. Scriven, BSc, PhD
Medical & Molecular Genetics, King's College London Medical School, Cytogenetics, 5th Floor, Tower Wing, Guy's Hospital, Great Maze Pond, London SE1 9RT, UK
e-mail: paul.scriven@kcl.ac.uk

T. El-Toukhy, P. Braude (eds.), *Preimplantation Genetic Diagnosis in Clinical Practice*, DOI 10.1007/978-1-4471-2948-6_11, © Springer-Verlag London 2014

121

What Data Are Available and How Valuable Are They?

PGD data is available in a number of different formats. Published data comprises centre-specific data, voluntary multicentric data collection, case reports and series as well as data from reference diagnostic laboratories. In addition, the mandatory data collected by some regulatory bodies is wholly web based, e.g. the HFEA. The inconsistency of collection and presentation makes it difficult to compare data sets between different centres and between countries (Table 11.1).

Understanding PGD Data

In order to understand and compare PGD outcome data, it is necessary to properly understand how routine IVF data is presented since PGD reflects a specialised IVF subgroup with added levels of complexity. The Human Fertilisation and Embryology Authority website provides an excellent basic guide to understanding IVF data. It is essential that the same terms and denominators used in routine non-PGD IVF are used when attempting to understand, collate and compare PGD outcome datasets particularly from different sources.

In order to capture relevant data, it is important to understand factors that can affect PGD outcome; those relating to fertility, which will affect IVF outcome in general, and those related to the specific genetic condition under investigation. Most PGD patients are not infertile; many present with affected children or have terminated affected pregnancies. However, their outcomes are still governed by the same factors that influence routine (non-PGD) IVF cycles, of which female age remains the single most important prognostic indicator of success. Younger age is closely associated with better oocyte (hence embryo) quality and numbers. For this reason any data set must account for such differences between patients and are best presented in age cohorts. The type of genetic condition for which PGD is offered is relevant

TABLE 11.1 Examples of published PGD (and PGS) data reports

Publication	Description	Strengths	Weaknesses
Harper et al. (2012)	ESHRE PGD Consortium data (10 years)	Good overview	Unverified
		Large data set	Partially validated
		Multiple centres	Voluntary submission
		Different countries	Limited analysis
		Very detailed information	Not all centres represented
Kuliev and Verlinsky (2004)	Large number of cycles from leading PGD centres	Multiple centres	Overlapping with other data sets
		International	Limited analysis
		Follow-up included	
Grace et al. (2006)	First 330 cycles at a UK centre	Unselected (consecutive)	Single centre
		Detailed information	Limited numbers (not generalisable)
			Historic data
de Die-Smulders et al. (2004)	First 100 cycles in the Netherlands	Unselected (consecutive)	Limited numbers (not generalisable)
		Detailed information	Historic data published in Dutch
HFEA (2013)	UK's mandatory data collection (for IVF and PGD)	Verified and validated data	Too little detail
		Patient friendly	No subcategorisation (e.g. biopsy method, inheritance, test method)
		Explanatory guide	Not PGD specific
Gutiérrez-Mateo et al. (2009)	Reference diagnostic laboratory	Comprehensive and detailed	IVF detail may be inaccurate/missing
		Multiple centres	
Wilton et al. (2009)	Misdiagnosis reports	Detailed analysis of cases	Self-reporting
			Likely underestimate

since the probability of having at least one unaffected embryo for transfer is based primarily on the mode of inheritance of the condition or an estimated risk of unbalanced gametes for a particular chromosomal translocation. Fewer embryos will be available for transfer when undertaking PGD for a dominant condition (e.g. Huntington's disease) in which an average 50 % of embryos are affected compared to a recessive condition (e.g. cystic fibrosis) in which only 25 % of embryos are affected. Since embryos within the same cohort have different implantation potentials, the larger the group of unaffected embryos available the higher the likelihood of selecting a viable embryo. Recent data from the ESHRE PGD Consortium illustrate these principles. A comparison of nearly 1,000 cycles demonstrated a higher rate of clinical pregnancies per egg retrieval and cycles reaching embryo transfer for autosomal recessive cycles compared with autosomal dominant cycles, but the implantation rate, a measure of the intrinsic embryo quality, was no different.

What Is the Expectation of Success Between PGD and Routine Non-PGD IVF Cycles?

It is difficult to reliably compare these two treatment modalities since it is uncommon for PGD patients to undergo IVF without PGD, and there are no well-controlled trial data available. Data from PGS trials and frozen embryo implantation data suggest a detrimental effect of embryo biopsy on both survival and implantation potential. In addition, the reduced number of embryos available for transfer after genetic selection compared with conventional IVF/ICSI also decreases likelihood of pregnancy. However, these negative factors are balanced to an unknown extent by the fact that most PGD patients do not have fertility problems. Taking into account these factors and the variety of the different indications for PGD, patients can be reassured that PGD success rates overall appear to be at least as good as those obtained in routine IVF/ICSI cycles (see Table 11.2).

Table 11.2 Cumulative 3-year HFEA data to end Q4 2010 (Age 35–37, fresh transfers, own eggs)

Centre	PGD (all indications)			IVF+ICSI (no-PGD)		
	ET cycles	Live births	LB (%)	ET cycles	Live births	LB (%)
A	102	39	38.2	884	287	32.5
B	6	0	0.0	719	339	47.1
C	10	3	30.0	984	368	37.4
D	5	3	60.0	684	275	40.2
E	34	16	47.1	401	180	44.9
F	2	0	0.0	443	175	39.5
G	6	1	16.7	556	152	27.3
H	1	0	0.0	1,151	333	28.9
I	2	0	0.0	1,043	363	34.8
Total	168	62	36.9 %	6,865	2,472	36.0 %

Analysis of Data

Understandably, the publication of centre-specific outcome data quickly can lead to the production of 'league tables' in which patients may search for the table-topping clinic(s). Such 'league tables' do not provide a comprehensive picture and can be misleading for patients for a number of reasons:

- Clinics may treat different patient populations.
- Clinics may be selective in which patients are treated.
- Most clinics carry out too few cycles annually to reliably predict general success.
- Live-birth rates reflect treatment carried out up to 2 years prior to data publication and may not accurately reflect a specific clinic's current practice.

However, the creation of anonymised league tables (Fig. 11.1) can be an excellent tool for benchmarking as part of continuous improvement, i.e. to enable centres to set aspirational targets of what is possible and thus drive best practice.

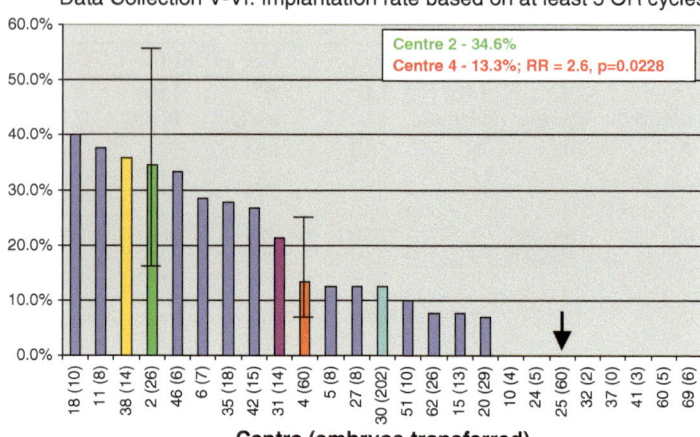

FIGURE 11.1 Illustration of detailed analysis made to compare implantation rates from PGD cycles for reciprocal translocations performed at different centres as a measure of IVF quality. All data abstracted from raw reciprocal translocation data provided during ESHRE PGD Consortium data collection V–VI. *X*-axis: number outside of parentheses indicates anonymised centre number. Number within parentheses indicates the number of embryos transferred. Implantation rate = total number fetal hearts/total number of embryos transferred. The *arrow* indicates that centre 25 transferred 60 embryos and none implanted

What We Have Learned from Published PGD Data

PGD cycle data have been collected and published at the individual clinic level, national and international level (in the form of working groups or consortia) with varying levels of success (Table 11.1). The advantage of individual clinic reports is the integrity of data; the drawback being that the small sample size prevents generalisable conclusions. In contrast, consortia data is based on large numbers of cycles reported from a wide range of centres, making the outcomes more generalisable; however, reporting an average may smooth differences between 'successful and unsuccessful' centres. The ideal data set would include enough cycles to be statistically robust but with a sufficient level of specific information to allow one to compare centres. The use of confidence intervals, ranges and graphical representations (e.g. funnel plots) can illustrate clearly how centres' success rates compare against the average while taking into account their cycle volume and thus the robustness of their results. The use of clinical pregnancies as well as live births using both cycle started and embryo transfer procedure as the denominator adds to robustness and transparency. The HFEA has recently provided not only the most up-to-date outcomes but also those from treatment cycles started in the three previous years to illustrate clinic consistency.

Future Opportunities

While enormous efforts have been made to collect, analyse and publish data from large numbers of cycles from multiple centres *voluntarily* reporting data (e.g. nearly 30,000 cycles were reported recently representing the first 10 years of data collection from the ESHRE PGD Consortium), it remains difficult to draw detailed conclusions from these data. Their main value appears to be threefold. First, they have provided an indication of cycle volumes year on year, the growth of PGD (and PGS) globally, crude success rates and the number of centres reporting data. Second, these data report misdiagnoses and perinatal outcomes providing a more 'warts and all' overview. Finally, these reports have been useful in describing trends in the evolution of PGD with respect to the adoption of specific techniques including laser-assisted biopsy, polar body and trophectoderm biopsy, new strategies, methodologies and technologies for diagnosis (e.g. microarrays) and the more frequent use and success of freezing biopsied embryos. More in-depth analysis by commentators using the raw data tables provided demonstrates a wide variation in the success rates between different centres (Fig. 11.1) supporting the need for greater standardisation and the principle that PGD should only be undertaken at IVF centres with a solid and successful routine IVF track record.

To ensure reliability of data requires *mandatory* reporting with verification and validation procedures in place. Such systems already exist in a number of countries (including the UK and the USA). The simplest, most efficient and least error-prone method of capturing such data would be to use a centralised online database to incorporate specific data fields from contributors using verified data with a comprehensive set of strict validation rules to prevent simple data entry errors. Such a database could be used to link with other international databases involving different areas of healthcare (e.g. cancer registry in order to identify possible links between IVF, PGD and cancer). Raw data should be available to researchers to facilitate additional analysis. Clearly these recommendations are aspirational and require vast amounts of resource, funding and international co-operation. Without pressure from governments and regulatory bodies, stringent data collection and submission will remain recommended best practice rather a mandatory activity.

Using Data to Choose a Clinic

For those wishing to refer patients or looking to purchase cycles of PGD, a number of different factors should be considered when assessing the suitability of a PGD centre or provider. Assuming large enough numbers are available to make meaningful comparisons, the success rates of PGD cycles overall should be assessed against the routine (non-PGD) cycles. If there are too few to assess for the most recent year, consider cumulative data from several years as reported by the HFEA (Table 11.2).

While data on pregnancy rates are an obvious and important index, there are other critical areas that should be assessed in choosing a suitable PGD service including: the clinic's overall experience and caseload, the ready availability of professional genetic counselling and advice, whether the PGD test is performed in-house or outsourced and the quoted accuracy of the test estimated following both valida-tion and clinical experience. A well-designed PGD test should aim to have as low risk of misdiagnosis as possible (<1 %), in order to be effective in preventing affected off-spring and the associated lifetime costs. Purchasers and refer-rers should ask about a centre's misdiagnosis rates and their experience and methods of handling adverse incidents as these are frequently under-reported. Finally, comprehensive written patient information should be readily available to patients and should be seen to properly deliver the information described above.

Key Points
- Current PGD data collections are of limited use either because of small sample size or lack of verification.
- Results reported in the literature generally are not verified or validated by an independent body nor do they represent a complete picture of PGD worldwide.
- Mandatory data collection would provide the most robust and reliable data for analysis.
- When comparing data sets, compare like with like. Not all 'success rates' are equivalent. For example, 'clinical pregnancy per cycle started' is not the same as 'live birth per embryo transfer'.
- Standardised nomenclature, outcomes and statistical analysis of data will help patients and providers make meaningful comparisons between PGD centres.
- Future databases should be able to link with existing medical databases (e.g. cancer registry) to identify any possible links between PGD and unrelated health outcomes.

- Careful counselling is required for all couples prior to starting a PGD cycle so that they understand the likely chances of success given their previous history, age, aetiology, PGD indication, treatment centre and so on.
- An individual clinic's caseload, laboratory experience, availability of genetic services, patient information and honesty about misdiagnosis rate is important in addition to success rate data in choosing an effective service.

Further Reading

Baruch S, Adamson GD, Cohen J, Gibbons WE, Hughes MR, Kuliev A, Munné S, Rebar RW, Simpson JL, Verlinsky Y, Hudson KL. Genetic testing of embryos: a critical need for data. Reprod Biomed Online. 2005;11(6):667–70.

de Die-Smulders CE, Land JA, Dreesen JC, Coonen E, Evers JL, Geraedts JP. Results from 10 years of preimplantation-genetic diagnostics in The Netherlands. Ned Tijdschr Geneeskd. 2004;148(50):2491–6.

Eshre PGD Consortium Steering Committee. ESHRE Preimplantation Genetic Diagnosis (PGD) consortium: preliminary assessment of data from January 1997 to September 1998. Hum Reprod. 1999; 14:3138–48.

Ferraretti AP, Goossens V, de Mouzon J, Bhattacharya S, Castilla JA, Korsak V, Kupka M, Nygren KG, Nyboe Andersen A,. The European IVF-monitoring (EIM); Consortium, for the European Society of Human Reproduction and Embryology (ESHRE). Assisted reproductive technology in Europe, 2008: results generated from European registers by ESHRE. Hum Reprod. 2012;27(9):2571–84.

Goossens V, Traeger-Synodinos J, Coonen E, De Rycke M, Moutou C, Pehlivan T, Derks-Smeets IA, Harton G. ESHRE PGD consortium data collection XI: cycles from January to December 2008 with pregnancy follow-up to October 2009. Hum Reprod. 2012;27(7):1887–911.

Grace J, El-Toukhy T, Scriven P, et al. Three hundred and thirty cycles of preimplantation genetic diagnosis for serious genetic disease: clinical considerations affecting outcome. Br J Obstet Gynaecol. 2006;113:1393–401.

Gutiérrez-Mateo C, Sánchez-García JF, Fischer J, Tormasi S, Cohen J, Munné S, Wells D. Preimplantation genetic diagnosis of single-gene disorders: experience with more than 200 cycles conducted by a reference laboratory in the United States. Fertil Steril. 2009; 92(5):1544–56.

Harper JC, Wilton L, Traeger-Synodinos J, Goossens V, Moutou C, SenGupta SB, Pehlivan Budak T, Renwick P, De Rycke M, Geraedts JP, Harton G. The ESHRE PGD consortium: 10 years of data collection. Hum Reprod Update. 2012;18(3):234–47.

Harton G, Braude P, Lashwood A, Schmutzler A, Traeger-Synodinos J, Wilton L, Harper JC,. European Society for Human Reproduction and Embryology (ESHRE) PGD Consortium. ESHRE PGD consortium best practice guidelines for organization of a PGD centre for PGD/preimplantation genetic screening. Hum Reprod. 2011;26(1):14–24.

HFEA. HFEA guide to understanding success rates. URL at 30th Apr 2013. http://www.hfea.gov.uk/fertility-clinics-success-rates.html.

Kuliev A, Verlinsky Y. Thirteen years' experience of preimplantation diagnosis: report of the fifth international symposium on preimplantation genetics. Reprod Biomed Online. 2004;8(2):229–35.

Wilton L, Thornhill A, Traeger-Synodinos J, Sermon KD, Harper JC. The causes of misdiagnosis and adverse outcomes in PGD. Hum Reprod. 2009;24(5):1221–8.

Chapter 12
PGD Facts and Figures

Tarek El-Toukhy

The first attempt at performing preimplantation genetic diagnosis at the PGD Centre at Guy's and St. Thomas' Hospital was in 1997 to select female embryos for a couple at risk of conceiving a child affected with X-linked haemophilia A, while the first live birth was achieved in a cycle performed in 1998 for spinal muscular atrophy (SMA) using a polymerase chain reaction (PCR)-based test. The PGD programme has progressively grown over time, such that the number of PGD cycles performed annually has increased from 50 cycles in 2000 to over 220 cycles in 2012 (Fig. 12.1), making it one of the largest PGD centres in Europe.

The main indications for PGD in our centre are (1) monogenic (autosomal dominant or recessive) disorders, (2) X-linked conditions and (3) chromosomal rearrangements. Approximately 60 % of PGD cycles use preimplantation genetic haplotyping (PGH) for monogenic disorders and 40 % use FISH for chromosomal rearrangements or embryo sexing for X-linked conditions. The two most common

T. El-Toukhy, MBBCh, MSc, MD, MRCOG
Assisted Conception Unit and PGD Centre, Guy's and St. Thomas' Hospital NHS Foundation Trust, 11th Floor, Tower Wing, Guy's Hospital, Great Maze Pond, London SE1 9RT, UK
e-mail: tarek.el-toukhy@gstt.nhs.uk

T. El-Toukhy, P. Braude (eds.), *Preimplantation Genetic Diagnosis in Clinical Practice*, DOI 10.1007/978-1-4471-2948-6_12, © Springer-Verlag London 2014

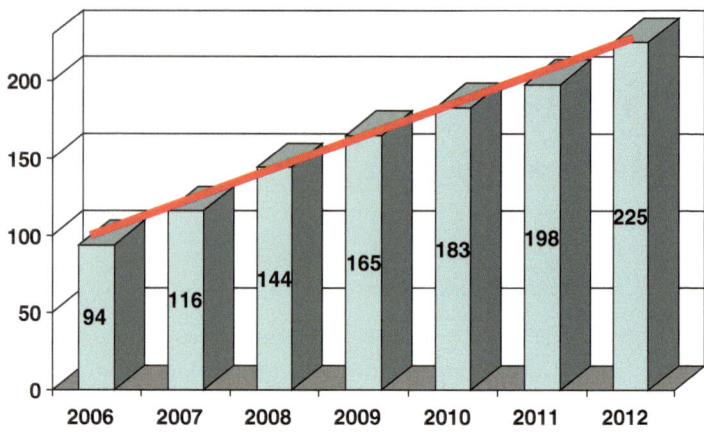

FIGURE 12.1 Number of PGD cycles started per year at the PGD Centre, Guy's and St. Thomas' Hospital NHS Foundation Trust

indications for PGD using PGH in our programme are cystic fibrosis and Huntington disease. Together they accounted for nearly 70 % of all PGD cycles performed for monogenic disorders between 2008 and 2012. Reciprocal chromosomal translocations accounted for 75 % of the indications for the use of FISH during the same period.

Outcome of PGD Cycles at GSTT

The average age of women starting a PGD cycle in our centre is 34 years. About 90 % of PGD cycles reach embryo biopsy, and 71 % reach embryo transfer. The latter figure is closely related to the type of genetic condition for which the embryos are tested. Carriers of reciprocal chromosomal translocations have the lowest likelihood of transfer due to the randomness of the meiotic chromosomal segregation outcomes (Table 12.1).

TABLE 12.1 Success rate per PGD cycle according to indication for PGD at the PGD Centre, Guy's and St. Thomas' Hospital NHS Foundation Trust (GSTT), 1,487 sequential cycles of PGD performed since 1998

	Single gene	X-linked	Rearrangements	Total
Cycles started	754	115	618	1,487
Cycles to retrieval	698	98	574	1,370
Cycles to biopsy	664	93	524	1,281
Cycles to transfer	583	85	387	1,055 (71 %)
Clinical pregnancy	249	31	152	432
Per retrieval (%)	36	31	26	32
Per transfer (%)	43	37	39	41

The mean number of oocytes retrieved is 12. On average, 6 embryos are biopsied and 4 out of 10 of these are transferable. Approximately half of the cycles reaching embryo transfer will have one or two embryos with a genetically transferable result, the other half having more than two. Two thirds of cycles reaching embryo transfer will have a single embryo replaced, and in over half of those transfers this will be done electively (i.e. in presence of more than one embryo suitable for transfer). In addition, a third of cycles reaching embryo transfer will have surplus embryos suitable for cryopreservation, currently performed via the vitrification method.

Overall, the clinical pregnancy rate per PGD cycle started is 29 %, per egg retrieval is 32 % and per embryo transfer is 41 %, although these figures will vary according to the indication for PGD treatment (Table 12.1).

Factors Affecting PGD Outcome

Female Age

Data from our programme show that women below 38 years of age are more than twice as likely to achieve a clinical pregnancy after a PGD cycle compared with older women (29 % vs. 13 %, OR = 2.8, 95 % CI 1.7–4.6, $P < 0.001$, respectively). This is related directly to increased embryo availability, improved embryo quality and lower risk of miscarriage in the younger age group.

Ovarian Reserve and Availability of Transferable Embryos

PGD cycles in which there are eight or more fertilised oocytes available are significantly more likely to lead to a clinical pregnancy (37 % vs. 21 %, OR = 2.2, 95 % CI 1.6–3.0, $P < 0.001$). This is due to the increased chance of reaching embryo transfer (90 % vs. 68 %, $P < 0.001$) and underscores the significant attrition process that occurs in PGD cycles as a result of embryo genetic testing. Furthermore, cycles in which there are surplus embryos available for cryopreservation significantly increases the chance of a clinical pregnancy in the fresh PGD cycle compared with cycles in which there are no surplus embryos available (52 % vs. 29 %, OR = 1.9, 95 % CI 1.3–2.9, $P = 0.0012$), probably because of superior embryo quality in the former scenario.

Type of Genetic Condition Being Tested

PGD cycles performed for chromosomal rearrangements have the lowest proportion of embryos genetically suitable for transfer (26 %), compared with X-linked and monogenic conditions (34 and 54 %, respectively). Therefore, these cycles are the least likely to reach embryo transfer (two thirds

TABLE 12.2 Comparison of the outcome of PGD and conventional IVF/ICSI cycles performed at GSTT

	PGD	IVF/ICSI
No. of cycles	826	4,150
No. of embryo transfers	578	3,532
No. of clinical pregnancies	212 (37 % per transfer)	1,216 (35 % per transfer)
Implantation rate	33 %	27 %

of cycles started) compared with X-linked and monogenic conditions (three quarters of cycles started). As a result, PGD cycles performed for chromosomal rearrangements have a lower success rate per PGD cycle started and per egg collection compared with X-linked and monogenic conditions, although this difference almost disappears when the success rate is calculated per embryo transfer (Table 12.1) because of similar embryo implantation potential.

Is There a Difference Between PGD and IVF/ICSI Success Rates?

A possible detrimental effect of embryo biopsy on its survival and implantation potential has been a concern. In order to investigate this possibility, we compared the outcome of PGD cycles performed since 1998 with that of over 4,000 conventional in vitro fertilisation (IVF) and intracytoplasmic sperm injection (ICSI) cycles performed between July 2004 and March 2009. Despite a reduced number of embryos available for PGD transfer compared with conventional IVF/ICSI, due to the additional selection undertaken on the basis of genetic analysis, our results show comparable implantation and clinical pregnancy rates per embryo transfer between the two groups. This would argue against a detrimental effect of the cleavage stage biopsy procedure on the development of preimplantation embryos (Table 12.2).

Blastocyst Cryopreservation and Reducing the Multiple Pregnancy Rate After PGD

Attempts to increase the chance of pregnancy in PGD cycles by replacing more than one embryo have led to a high multiple pregnancy rate, which now represents the single most significant iatrogenic complication of assisted reproductive technology, including PGD. According to the ESHRE PGD Consortium data, about 40 % of babies born after PGD treatment were part of a multiple pregnancy. Indeed, multiple pregnancy after PGD treatment is even more problematic than after conventional IVF because of the possible need for prenatal testing and the effect of a multiple birth on caring for the existing family (Chap. 3).

In conventional IVF/ICSI cycles, elective single blastocyst transfer (SBT) followed by transfer of cryo-thawed blastocysts later if necessary has yielded high pregnancy rates. However, as similar strategy has not been widely adopted in PGD cycles because of concern about the reduced number of transferable embryos following biopsy and diagnosis.

From January 2006, all couples in our centre who had two or more disease-free transferable PGD blastocysts on day 5 of in vitro culture were offered SBT and cryopreservation of supernumerary blastocyst(s) for their future use. Adopting this policy has enabled our centre to reduce the multiple pregnancy rate in the PGD programme from 38 % before 2006 to 10 % thereafter (OR = 0.20, 95 % CI 0.08–0.48, $P < 0.001$) without any reduction in the success rate of the fresh PGD cycles or the overall cumulative ongoing pregnancy rate in our programme. We have also demonstrated that the survival and implantation potential of biopsied PGD embryos cryopreserved at the blastocyst stage using a slow-freezing protocol is comparable to that of non-biopsied IVF/ICSI cryopreserved blastocysts. Between 2006 and 2012, we performed 179 frozen-thawed embryo transfer cycles using thawed PGD embryos, achieving a pregnancy rate of 42 % and clinical pregnancy rate of 26 % per thaw, and a multiple pregnancy rate of 7 % per clinical pregnancy.

Key Points
- Single-gene disorders represent 60 % of the current indications for PGD.
- Approximately three quarters of PGD cycles started will reach embryo transfer.
- About 40 % of PGD embryo transfers will result in a clinical pregnancy.
- Female age and ovarian reserve are strong predictors of PGD success.
- Single blastocyst transfer and cryopreservation of surplus blastocyst(s) is an effective strategy to reduce the multiple pregnancy rate in a PGD programme.

Further Reading

El-Toukhy T, Kamal A, Wharf E, et al. Reduction of the multiple pregnancy rate in a preimplantation genetic diagnosis programme after introduction of single blastocyst transfer and cryopreservation of blastocysts biopsied on day 3. Hum Reprod. 2009;24:2642–8.

Grace J, El-Toukhy T, Scriven P, et al. Three hundred and thirty cycles of preimplantation genetic diagnosis for serious genetic disease: clinical considerations affecting outcome. Br J Obstet Gynaecol. 2006;113: 1393–401.

Harper J, Wilton L, Traeqer-Synodinos J, et al. The ESHRE PGD consortium: 10 years of data collection. Hum Reprod Update. 2012;18: 234–47.

Pickering S, Polidoropoulos N, Caller J, et al. Preimplantation Genetic Diagnosis Study Group. Strategies and outcomes of the first 100 cycles of preimplantation genetic diagnosis at the Guy's and St. Thomas' Center. Fertil Steril. 2003;79:81–90.

Chapter 13
Preimplantation Genetic Diagnosis and HLA-Typing: The Potential for Selection of Unaffected HLA Matched Siblings

Lucie Brown and H. Bobby Gaspar

Bone marrow transplantation, or more correctly haematopoietic stem cell transplantation (HSCT), is an effective treatment for many disorders of the haematopoietic system. HSCT involves taking haematopoietic stem cells from a healthy donor and transferring them into an affected individual such that the recipient forms a new haematopoietic system that is free of disease. Although HSCT is most commonly used for haematological malignancies (acute and

L. Brown, BSc, Children's Nursing (✉)
Department of Immunology and Bone Marrow Transplant,
Paediatric Nurse Practitioner-Immunology and Bone Marrow
Transplant, Great Ormond Street Hospital for Children NHS
Foundation Trust, Great Ormond Street Hospital,
Great Ormond Street, London WC1N 3JH, UK
e-mail: lucinda.brown@gosh.nhs.uk

H.B. Gaspar, MBBS, MRCP(UK), MRCPCH, PhD
Molecular Immunology Unit, Great Ormond Street Hospital
and UCL Institute of Child Health, 30, Guilford Street,
London WC1N, UK
e-mail: h.gaspar@ucl.ac.uk

T. El-Toukhy, P. Braude (eds.), *Preimplantation Genetic
Diagnosis in Clinical Practice*, DOI 10.1007/978-1-4471-2948-6_13,
© Springer-Verlag London 2014

chronic leukaemias and lymphomas), it is also used increasingly for the treatment of severe immunodeficiencies, specific metabolic diseases and haemoglobinopathies such as β-thalassaemia major and sickle-cell anaemia. If effective, HSCT has the potential to offer a cure for life and is therefore an extremely important treatment option and for some genetic conditions the only option available. The success of transplant is influenced by many factors but most importantly by the availability of a well-matched healthy donor to provide the source of donor stem cells. Numerous reports show that the best survival outcomes are achieved when a sibling who has the same genetic HLA type as the patient is available.

PGD has the ability to identify many genetic characteristics of the embryo, including importantly the HLA type. For that reason, there has been increasing interest in the use of PGD techniques to select embryos that not only are genetically unaffected but are also an HLA match for older siblings who require a HSCT. The use of PGD and HLA typing is at present limited with just a handful of centres offering this service, and there have been few reports of successful births using this approach although the numbers are increasing. However, as the technology becomes more widely available, it is likely that PGD combined with HLA typing will be used to select healthy donors for a number of genetic disorders. This chapter will explain in more detail what HLA typing involves and the specific conditions where it may be applicable.

What Is HLA Typing?

The human histocompatibility complex (HLA) is positioned on the short arm of chromosome 6 (Fig. 13.1). The HLA loci are part of the genetic region known as the major histocompatibility complex (MHC) which is fundamental for normal function and regulation of the immune response. The HLA complex is critical for the immune system to distinguish self from nonself, thus providing protection against invading microorganisms. The molecules encoded by the HLA genes present foreign proteins

Chromosome 6

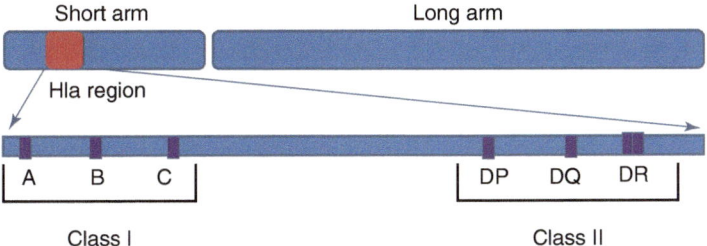

FIGURE 13.1 HLA region on chromosome 6p21.3 (Representation of the HLA locus on chromosome 6 and the distribution of the Class I and II genes)

to effector immune cells, which can then identify each cell of the body as its own and reject or kill infected or foreign cells.

The HLA system has been described as the most polymorphic genetic structure in humans and demonstrates significant differences in the amino acid sequences of HLA-encoded MHC proteins between individuals. The term tissue type or HLA type is the term used to describe the HLA genetic make-up of any individual; tissue typing or HLA typing refers to the process of determining the HLA type. When searching for a matched donor for HSCT, the goal is to find an individual who has the same HLA type as the recipient.

The HLA System Comprises of Two Classes: HLA Class I and Class II

HLA Class I molecules are expressed on the surface of almost all nucleated cells and are known as HLA-A, HLA-B and HLA-C genes. Class II antigens, HLA-DR, HLA-DQ and HLA-DP, are only expressed on the surface of B lymphocytes, monocytes and T lymphocytes that are involved in the immune response. These 6 loci, called A, B, C, DQ, DR and

DP, are what are normally referred to when discussing HLA matching in the context of HSCT, although in most cases the DP loci are not routinely used. At each locus, there is considerable variability in the genetic sequences that have been inherited through evolution. Thus, there are numerous HLA-A alleles, each of which is given a specific nomenclature (A*0101, A*0201, A*0202, etc.). The HLA types can also be recognised by serotherapy, i.e. by the use of antibodies directed against the antigens expressed by the alleles; thus, nearly all HLA*A0101 alleles are recognised by HLA-A1 antibody, and 75 % of HLA-A*0103 are recognised by HLA-A1. Allelic DNA typing will give the most definitive tissue type and is the only way HLA typing can be performed for PGD. Specific genes are more common within certain populations.

Why Is HLA Typing Important in HSCT?

Any cell with a different HLA type to the host is recognised by the host immune system as nonself, resulting in the destruction or rejection of the tissue with those cells. In the context of haematopoietic stem cell transplantation (HSCT), donor's cells may be recognised as nonself and be rejected by the host. Conversely, engrafted donor T cells may recognise the host tissues as being foreign, therefore attacking vital organs. This process is known as graft versus host disease and is the most common and most severe complication following HSCT. The greater the disparity of HLA matching between the patient and donor, the higher the risk of transplant-related mortality (TRM) as a result of these described complications.

HLA Matched Donors

Each individual has two different HLA haplotypes; one set of HLA antigens is inherited from each parent (Fig. 13.2). Therefore, two siblings who inherit the same two HLA haplotypes from their parents will be HLA identical, and

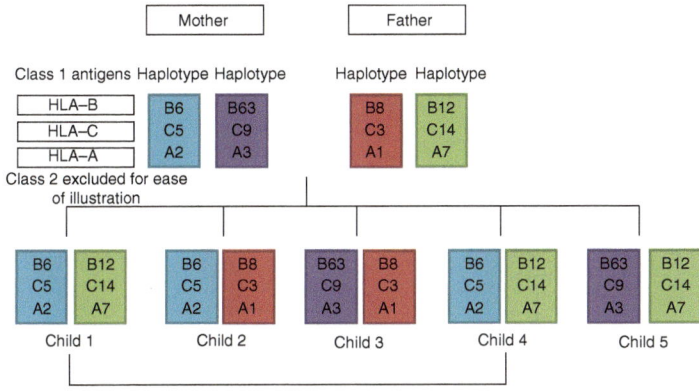

FIGURE 13.2 Inheritance of HLA antigens. HLA genes are inherited in a linked manner and in a conventional autosomal pattern. Thus, there is a 1:4 chance of two siblings sharing the same HLA type. For ease of illustration, only the inheritance of Class I genes is shown in this diagram, but Class II genes are inherited in an identical way

given normal autosomal inheritance, there is a 1 in 4 chances that this will occur.

Numerous studies have shown that a transplant from an HLA identical sibling results in the best survival outcomes. The figures vary for different diseases. For example, in HSCT for severe immune deficiencies, long-term survival following a matched sibling donor transplant is 71 % in comparison to 63 % survival from a matched unrelated donor or 39 % survival from a mismatched donor (Fig. 13.3). An HLA identical sibling donor therefore gives the best possible chance of survival. Unfortunately, only approximately one third of children requiring a stem cell transplant have an HLA identical sibling.

In the absence of an HLA identical sibling, a volunteer unrelated donor search is initiated through bone marrow transplant registries. Allele compatibility for the HLA-A/B/C/DRB1/DQB1 loci is defined as 10/10 match and is the favoured level of matching when considering an unrelated donor for stem cell transplantation. The number of donors joining bone marrow

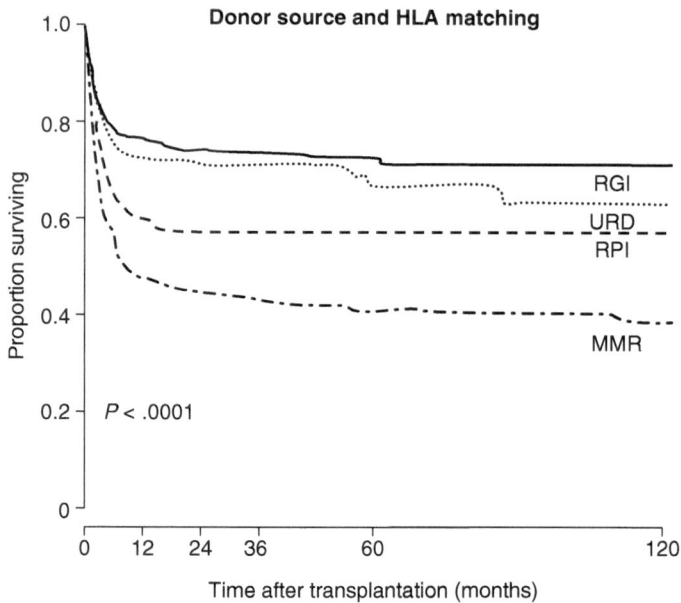

RGI- related genotypical identical donor (matched sibling donor)
URD- unrelated donor
RPI- related phenotypical identical donor (matched family donor)
MMR -mismatched related donor

FIGURE 13.3 Outcome following different donor transplants for non-SCID T cell immunodeficiencies. The importance of donor matching is shown in this figure. The best survival figures are seen after transplant from a related genotypically identical (*RGI*) donor which is normally a matched sibling. Outcomes following transplant from other donor sources are less good

registries continues to grow worldwide. This, along with the use of umbilical cord blood as an additional source of haematopoietic stem cells, has increased the chance of finding a matched unrelated donor. However, as the survival figures demonstrate, a matched unrelated donor transplant is less successful than a sibling donor transplant, and this results from differences at minor histocompatibility antigens as well as other factors.

Indications for Preimplantation HLA Matching

Simply put, the indications for PGD with HLA matching are that the patient must lack a well-matched family, unrelated or umbilical cord donor. However, exact criteria are more difficult to define and will vary with the disease, the type of donor available, the reported outcomes available from different donor sources and family and physician preferences. For example, for a given disease, one centre may feel comfortable with proceeding with a 1 antigen mismatched umbilical donor transplant. By contrast, if this was the only donor available and there was limited experience of umbilical cord procedures, another centre might decide with the family to proceed with PGD-HLA typing. Clearly, the exact molecular genetic basis for the disease would need to be known so that an unaffected embryo can be unambiguously selected.

Delays in Proceeding with PGD

Even following a decision to proceed with PGD with HLA, it can take a number of years for an unaffected compatible sibling to be born. It may well take up to a year before a couple can embark on their first cycle of PGD partly due to the time taken to secure funding from local primary care trusts, partly the time taken for disease specific assays to be developed in the PGD laboratory and time for fertility tests to be performed in the assisted conception unit.

The addition of HLA typing to embryo selection adds another layer of complexity to the procedure. Besides the technical developments required to perform multiplex PCR on single embryo cells to determine the HLA type, the search for an appropriate embryo may not always be successful. For a standard autosomal recessive condition, the statistics of generating an unaffected (3/4) and a HLA matched (1/4) embryo are 3/16. Thus, mothers may have to go through multiple stimulation cycles before an appropriate embryo is identified.

These delays make it essential that the clinical condition of the affected child is stable and can be maintained relatively so for a number of years until a matched sibling donor is generated. In the context of immunodeficiencies, this requirement would exclude conditions such as severe combined immunodeficiency where transplantation is recommended within months of diagnosis because of the risk of severe infections. However, other conditions such as Wiskott-Aldrich syndrome and chronic granulomatous disease, where patients can be placed on protective therapy and where deterioration of the condition is more insidious, could be considered suitable. For many metabolic diseases, there is an urgency to transplant early because of concerns regarding neurological deterioration. Conditions such as X-linked adrenoleukodystrophy where there is a more gradual onset may be more appropriate. Haemoglobinopathies and red cell disorders such as Diamond-Blackfan syndrome are possibly the most amenable to preimplantation HLA matching since patients can be maintained on red blood cell transfusions and iron chelation therapy for many years before definitive therapy is considered. Another possible indication is Fanconi's anaemia where bone marrow failure is most commonly seen in later rather than early childhood. A table of possible indications is given (Table 13.1).

Ethical Considerations

Testing the preimplantation embryo for genetic disease is done in the best interests of the embryo or the person it will become. However, it is argued that when embryo biopsy is performed for HLA typing alone, the only benefit is to the existing sick child. In the case of PGD with HLA typing, where the couple wish to expand their family by having an unaffected child and the opportunity exists for that child to also be an HLA match, these two indications are combined. Some argue that creating 'saviour siblings' is not creating a child in their own right but merely designing it for instrumental reasons to serve as a donor for the sick child.

TABLE 13.1 Possible indications for PGD and HLA typing

Disease types	Examples of specific disorders
Immune deficiencies	Wiskott-Aldrich syndrome
	Chronic granulomatous disease
	X-linked hyper IgM syndrome
	X-linked lymphoproliferative disease
	Leukocyte adhesion deficiency type I
Metabolic disorders	X-linked adrenoleukodystrophy
Haemoglobinopathies	Thalassaemias
	Sickle-cell disease
Red cell disorders	Diamond-Blackfan syndrome
Genetic disorders of bone marrow failure	Fanconi anaemia

The collection of stem cells from the HLA-matched sibling would be arranged through collecting and storing umbilical cord blood at birth. This technique can be arranged so as not to cause any harm to the mother or newborn child. Nevertheless, the procedure is not always successful as the required number of stem cells may not be collected via this method. This naturally leads to an important question: 'what may be done to the donor child in order to treat a sibling'. It has been argued that the standard employed in this situation is what is acceptable if the donor child already existed. Bone marrow harvests on sibling donors are a routine procedure, but any general anaesthetic and operative procedure still carries a small risk to the child.

Alternative Treatments Options and Their Availability

Definitive treatments for genetic disorders of the bone marrow are very limited. A number of possibilities for maintenance rather than cure are available, but often these do not correct the disease phenotype, and there is ongoing deterioration or organ damage. These include a number of enzyme replacement therapies for both immune deficiency and specific metabolic disorders. In addition to lack of full efficacy, these therapies can be extremely expensive. Gene therapy is now also being developed for genetic bone marrow disorders. This procedure involves extraction and genetic modification of the child's own bone marrow stem cells prior to reinfusion. By using the child's own cells, this has the benefit of not requiring a donor and avoiding the risk of graft versus host disease. Gene therapy has successfully corrected a number of immunodeficiencies and is in development for a range of metabolic disorders and haemoglobinopathies. Initial studies were complicated by development of leukaemias in treated patients as a result of the mode of gene delivery. A new wave of trials using modified delivery strategies are now underway. The wider applicability of gene therapy will be determined by the success or otherwise of these forthcoming clinical trials.

Key Points
- Preimplantation HLA typing provides the opportunity to select an HLA-matched unaffected embryo that may be a suitable HSCT donor for an affected sibling.
- A matched sibling donor is always a desired option and for specific families who wish to have another healthy child and who have a child with a later-onset disease; preimplantation HLA matching may be the treatment of choice.
- The time it takes to select and generate an appropriate donor means that it can only be useful for conditions that do not require transplant in near term.
- Currently facilities are limited and creating expertise in specific centres to offer improved access and availability of preimplantation HLA matching will increase uptake of this technology.
- Increasing the success of transplants from unrelated and mismatched donor transplants and the development of autologous haematopoietic stem cell gene therapy will provide increasing options for patients.

Further Reading

Devolder K. Preimplantation HLA typing: having children to save our loved ones. J Med Ethics. 2005;31:582–6.

El-Toukhy T, Bickerstaff H, Meller S. Preimplantation genetic diagnosis for haematologic conditions. Curr Opin Pediatr. 2010;22(1):28–34.

Gennery et al. J Allergy Clin Immunol. 2010;126(3):602–10.

Kahraman S, Beyazyurek C, Ekmekci CG. Seven years of experience of preimplantation HLA typing: a clinical overview of 327 cycles. Reprod Biomed Online. 2011;23(3):363–71.

Ljungman P, Bregni M, Brune M, European Group for Blood and Marrow Transplantation, et al. Allogeneic and autologous transplantation for haematological diseases, solid tumours and immune disorders: current practice in Europe 2009. Bone Marrow Transplant. 2010; 45(2):219–34.

Pennings G, Schots R, Liebaers I. Ethical considerations on preimplantation genetic diagnosis for HLA typing to match a future child as a donor of haematopoietic stem cells to a sibling. Hum Reprod. 2002; 17:534–8.

Rivat C, Santilli G, Gaspar HB, Thrasher AJ. Gene therapy for primary immunodeficiencies. Hum Gene Ther. 2012;23(7):668–75. doi:10.1089/hum.2012.116.

Shankarkumar U. The human leukocyte antigen system (HLA) system. Int J Human Genet. 2004;4(2):91–103.

Zierhut H, MacMillan ML, Wagner JE, Bartels DM. More than 10 years after the first 'savior siblings': parental experiences surrounding preimplantation genetic diagnosis. J Genet Couns. 2013;22(5):594–602.

Chapter 14
PGD and Human Embryonic Stem Cell Technology

Emma Stephenson, Dusko Ilic, Laureen Jacquet, Olga Genbacev, and Susan J. Fisher

E. Stephenson, PhD • D. Ilic, MD, PhD (✉)
L. Jacquet, PhD student
Assisted Conception Unit, Guy's and St. Thomas
Hospital NHS Foundation Trust, 11th Floor, Tower Wing,
Great Maze Pond, London SE1 9RT, UK
e-mail: emma.stephenson@kcl.ac.uk;
dusko.ilic@kcl.ac.uk; laureen.jacquet@kcl.ac.uk

O. Genbacev, PhD
Division of Maternal Fetal Medicine, Department of Obstetrics,
Gynecology and Reproductive Sciences, University of California
San Francisco, The Eli and Edythe Broad Center for Regeneration
Medicine and Stem Cell Research, 35 Medical Center Way,
San Francisco 94143-0665, CA, USA
e-mail: genbacev@comcast.net

S.J. Fisher, PhD
Division of Maternal Fetal Medicine, Department of Obstetrics,
Gynecology and Reproductive Sciences, Sandler-Moore Mass
Spectrometry Core Facility, University of California San Francisco,
The Eli and Edythe Broad Center for Regeneration Medicine
and Stem Cell Research, 35 Medical Center Way, RMB-900H,
San Francisco 94143-0665, CA, USA
e-mail: sfisher@cgl.ucsf.edu

T. El-Toukhy, P. Braude (eds.), *Preimplantation Genetic*
Diagnosis in Clinical Practice, DOI 10.1007/978-1-4471-2948-6_14,
© Springer-Verlag London 2014

Human embryonic stem (hES) cells are derived from an early embryo and can grow in vitro indefinitely, while retaining their capability to differentiate into specialised somatic cell types. Two types of hES cells are being derived:

1. Those intended for clinical use in regenerative medicine
2. Those that carry disease-specific mutations and may serve as 'disease-in-a-dish' models

PGD technology was instrumental in the derivation of both types of hES cells.

Derivation of hES Cell Lines

The first reported hES cells were derived from blastocysts generated by in vitro fertilisation at the University of Wisconsin. By the end of 2009, nearly 1,200 original hES cell lines had been reported from 24 countries. Most of the lines were derived from the inner cell mass (ICM) of blastocyst stage embryos, employing a technology similar to the one developed by the group from Wisconsin. Reports that hES cells could be derived from the late morula/compaction stage and from cleavage stage embryos arrested in development demonstrated that pluripotent cells could give rise to hES cell lines at any stage of early embryo development.

hES cell culture is generally made up of two basic components – a fibroblast 'feeder' layer to which the hES cells attach and a specially designed culture medium which surrounds the cells as they grow. Within a stable temperature and gaseous environment, these components provide the cells with a scaffold to grow over and nutrients for growth, maintain an appropriate pH and, when optimal, support rapid undifferentiated proliferation. The exact details of these components vary across laboratories around the world, and differing levels of success are achieved in terms of derivation rates and cell line maintenance efficiency. The original culture systems used murine feeder cells and media based around fetal bovine serum. Most of the known hES cell lines have therefore been derived under conditions that expose the cells to products of animal origin, which renders them unsuitable for clinical use due to the risk of transmitting animal pathogens to recipients. Over time, however, the replacement of murine with human feeders and media based on bovine with defined culture media devoid of animal products has led to xeno-free derivation and expansion techniques for both research and clinical grade hES cell lines. As well as xeno-free derivation and propagation, stringent record-keeping, proof of sterility, negative virology and detailed characterisation of the cell lines are necessary to meet current clinical grade recommendations and good manufacturing practice (GMP) criteria, qualifying the cells for therapeutic use. Characterisation of the cells routinely includes DNA fingerprinting, HLA typing, karyotyping, expression of pluripotency markers and differentiation into derivatives of the three germ layers with in vitro expression of markers and in vivo teratoma growth.

Derivation of hES Cell Lines from a Single Blastomere

To avoid ethical and political controversies surrounding use of supernumerary embryos in research, efforts have been made to use alternative methods such as somatic cell nuclear transfer and parthenogenetic activation of human oocytes. However, neither of them has become a mainstream approach. The method that has become a popular option for circumventing political restrictions, particularly in the USA, is the derivation of hES cell lines from single cells of the cleavage stage embryo. Robert Lanza's group from the American company Advanced Cell Technology from Massachusetts (www.advancedcell.com) utilised a PGD technique to develop a groundbreaking approach to the derivation of hES cell lines using a single biopsied blastomere. Although the embryo was destroyed in the process, this was proof of principle that a hES cell line could be derived without embryo destruction. Indeed, in subsequent reports from the same group as well as others, the biopsied embryos survived and developed to the blastocyst stage. hES cell lines derived from a single blastomere exhibit very similar transcriptional profiles to hES cell lines derived from the ICM, suggesting that over time in culture hES cells acquire virtually identical stable phenotypes and are not affected by the developmental stage of the starting cell population.

One of the lines developed by Lanza's group from a single blastomere, MA-09, was used to develop an hES cell-based therapy, currently in clinical trials in multiple centres in the USA and UK, for the treatment of Stargardt's macular dystrophy and dry age-related macular degeneration.

Derivation of Specific Mutation-Carrying hES Cell Lines

Embryos diagnosed as being genetically unsuitable for replacement following PGD analysis would routinely be discarded, despite often being of good quality and capable of developing into blastocysts. With appropriate consent, these blastocysts are suitable for stem cell derivation and are free from many ethical difficulties associated with using normal embryos from patients seeking infertility treatment. With the fundamental attributes of pluripotency and self-renewal, hES cells carrying genetic disorders hold promise for an unlimited supply of cells with which to study the mechanisms and development of the disease. hES cells from PGD embryos should represent an even more relevant model than genetically altered cells or animal models as the mutant protein is expressed in its normal physiological context and range of expression pattern. The use of such 'disease-in-a-dish' models of genetic and degenerative disorders would also reduce the need for animal models. If highly purified colonies of known constituent cells can be developed through precise characterisation and sorting, they may prove useful in the long run, especially in terms of drug screening for new compounds and testing of unacceptable side effects. This could speed up the development to implementation process thus getting new drugs out more rapidly for use by the public. hES cell lines, particularly those carrying clinically relevant mutations, have gained considerable interest from the biopharmaceutical sector. The pharmaceutical discovery process is generally accepted as being time consuming and inefficient requiring high levels of financial investment without any guarantee of a clinical product at the end. Improvements to the discovery phase of new compounds could come through the development of more tailored, disease-orientated cellular screens, for both therapeutic target validation and optimisation of identified compounds.

hES cell lines have been derived with a number of monogenic disorders as well as disease-specific translocations (Tables 14.1 and 14.2). The largest number of PGD cell lines have been derived from embryos carrying a mutation for cystic fibrosis (22) and Huntington's disease (20). We have previously published our experience with the use of affected PGD embryos having derived the first hES cell line in the UK and the first line with a cystic fibrosis mutation. In addition we have now derived more than 20 hES cell lines carrying clinically relevant genetic mutations for eight monogenic diseases and one translocation (Table 14.3). The validation of hES cells as models of disease has begun for some disorders, including Huntington's disease, myotonic dystrophy and fragile X.

Induced Pluripotent Stem Cell Lines

In 2006, scientists found a way of reverting differentiated cells from adult mice into an embryonic-like state. In a groundbreaking publication, the following year Yamanaka and colleagues described the induction of pluripotent stem (iPS) cells from adult human fibroblasts by defined factors that are associated with the pluripotent state. These iPS cells were similar (but not identical) to hES cells in morphology,

TABLE 14.1 Specific mutation-carrying hES cell lines reported by May 17, 2012

Disease	Number of lines
Adrenoleukodystrophy	1
Albinism ocular, type1	2
Alpha-thalassaemia	2
Alport syndrome	2
Beta thalassaemia	6
Beta thalassaemia carrier	3
Breast cancer	2
Breast cancer and endocrine neoplasia	1
Charcot-Marie-Tooth disease, type 1A	3
Charcot-Marie-Tooth disease, type 1B	1
Cystic fibrosis	22
Cystic fibrosis carrier	1
Epidermolysis bullosa	1
Fabry syndrome	1
Fanconi anaemia – a carrier	1
Fragile site mental retardation 1, carrier	1
Fragile X syndrome	6
Fragile X syndrome, carrier	5
Gaucher disease	1
Haemoglobin alpha locus	1
Haemoglobin beta locus mutation	3
Haemophilia A	1
Huntington's disease	20
Huntington's disease and Marfan syndrome	1
Hypochondroplasia	1
Incontinentia pigmenti	1
Infantile neuroaxonal dystrophy	1
Juvenile retinoschisis	1

TABLE 14.1 (continued)

Disease	Number of lines
Marfan syndrome	3
Merosin-deficient congenital muscular dystrophy, type 1A	1
Multiple endocrine neoplasia, type 1	1
Multiple endocrine neoplasia, type 2	3
Muscular dystrophy, Becker	1
Muscular dystrophy, Becker, carrier	1
Muscular dystrophy, Duchenne	5
Muscular dystrophy, Duchenne, carrier	1
Muscular dystrophy, Emery-Dreifuss	1
Muscular dystrophy, Emery-Dreifuss, carrier	3
Muscular dystrophy, facioscapulohumeral	9
Muscular dystrophy, facioscapulohumeral and Turner syndrome	1
Muscular dystrophy, facioscapulohumeral, putative	2
Myotonic dystrophy	6
Myotonic dystrophy, type 1	4
Myotonic dystrophy, type 2	1
Nemaline myopathy 2	2
NEMO deficiency	2
Neurofibromatosis, type I	9
Osteogenesis imperfecta, type 1	1
Patau syndrome	1
Pelizaeus-Merzbacher disease	1
Popliteal pterygium syndrome	1
Saethre-Chotzen syndrome	1
Sandhoff disease	1
Sickle-cell anaemia	2

(continued)

TABLE 14.1 (continued)

Disease	Number of lines
Spinal muscular atrophy, type I	3
Spinocerebellar ataxia, type 2	1
Spinocerebellar ataxia, type 7	1
Torsion dystonia	1
Torsion dystonia 1	4
Translocation, 7:12	1
Translocation, 7:17	1
Translocation, 11:22	1
Treacher Collins-Franceschetti syndrome	2
Tuberous sclerosis, type 1	3
Turner syndrome, mosaic cell line	1
Vitelliform macular dystrophy	2
Von Hippel-Lindau disease	5
Wilms' tumour	1
Wiskott-Aldrich syndrome, cystic fibrosis carrier	1
X-linked myotubular myopathy	2
Zellweger syndrome	1

Strulovici et al. (2007), Löser et al. (2010); University of Massachusetts Medical School, International Stem Cell Registry http://www. umassmed.edu/iscr/GeneticDisorders.aspx; http://www.stemride. com/ accessed on May 17, 2012, including those derived at Assisted Conception Unit at Guy's Hospital as of May 17, 2012, sorted by disease type

proliferation, surface antigens, gene expression and differentiation ability. These cells are therefore as powerful as those isolated from early embryos and free of controversy. Since then, this new iPS cell field has enjoyed unprecedented popularity. Indeed all the advantages of using PGD hES cell lines as disease models also apply to the use of human iPS cells with the added attraction of a greater number of diseases,

TABLE 14.2 Specific mutation-carrying hES cell lines reported by May 17, 2012

Country	Number of lines
USA	91
Australia	32
UK	22
France	21
Israel	18
Belgium	16
Spain	1
Turkey	1
Total	202

Strulovici et al. (2007), Löser et al. (2010); University of Massachusetts Medical School, International Stem Cell Registry http://www.umassmed.edu/iscr/GeneticDisorders.aspx; http://www.stemride.com/ accessed on May 17, 2012, including those derived at Assisted Conception Unit at Guy's Hospital as of May 17, 2012, sorted by country of derivation

TABLE 14.3 Specific mutation-carrying hES cell lines derived at Assisted Conception Unit at Guy's Hospital as of May 17, 2012

Disease	Number of lines
Beta thalassaemia	1
Beta thalassaemia carrier	1
Cystic fibrosis	4
Huntington's disease	7
Myotonic dystrophy, type 1	1
Neurofibromatosis, type I	2
Spinal muscular atrophy, type I	1
Translocation, 7:12	1
Von Hippel-Lindau disease	3
Wiskott-Aldrich syndrome, cystic fibrosis carrier	1

easier availability of starting material, the use of samples from the diseased tissue and from donors in the age range when the disease occurs and fewer ethical issues. Furthermore stem cell models of some complex degenerative diseases such as Parkinson's, autism or Alzheimer's, for which no single predictive gene has been identified, will not be available through PGD but could be through the use of iPS technology.

Future Outlook

hES cells remain the only genetically unmodified pluripotent cells and as such remain the gold standard for pluripotency research. Research into the field of hES cells will continue in order to understand the basic mechanisms of pluripotency and self-renewal, as the gold standard with which to compare iPS cells; to investigate heterogeneity in pluripotent cells, as a powerful tool for modelling diseases; to investigate early human development; and because hES cells are years ahead of iPS cells in terms of safety for preclinical and clinical studies. Therefore the importance of PGD as a source of embryos for stem cell research is likely to grow. With the ever-increasing number of diseases for which PGD can be offered, and the continuous improvements to hES cell derivation and propagation methods, we anticipate that our bank of mutation-carrying hES cell lines will continue to grow rapidly, providing a unique and vital cell source that is freely available to researchers worldwide.

Key Points
- PGD technology has been instrumental in the derivation of both research and clinical grade human embryonic stem (hES) cell line.
- A line derived using the PGD technique of single blastomere biopsy is being used in the first clinical trial in Europe using hES cells and is the only currently ongoing clinical trial in the world.

- hES cell lines carrying clinically relevant genetic mutations are derived from affected embryos diagnosed in a PGD cycle and can be used as 'disease-in-a-dish' models.
- These PGD lines, in combination with induced pluripotent stem cell lines from affected patients, are a powerful tool for disease research.
- There is interest from the biopharmaceutical sector in the use of these mutation-carrying lines for drug discovery and toxicology screening.

Further Reading

Chung Y, Klimanskaya I, Becker S, Li T, Maserati M, Lu SJ, Zdravkovic T, Ilic D, Genbacev O, Fisher S, Krtolica A, Lanza R. Human embryonic stem cell lines generated without embryo destruction. Cell Stem Cell. 2008;2(2):113–7.

Franklin SB, Hunt C, Cornwell G, Peddie V, Desousa P, Livie M, Desousa P, Livie M, Stephenson EL, Braude PR. hESCCO: development of good practice models for hES cell derivation. Regen Med. 2008;3(1): 105–16.

Lei T, Jacob S, Ajil-Zaraa I, Dubuisson JB, Irion O, Jaconi M, Feki A. Xeno-free derivation and culture of human embryonic stem cells: current status, problems and challenges. Cell Res. 2007;17(8):682–8.

Löser P, Schirm J, Guhr A, Wobus AM, Kurtz A. Human embryonic stem cell lines and their use in international research. Stem Cells. 2010;28(2):240–6.

Sermon KD, Simon C, Braude P, Viville S, Borstlap J, Veiga A. Creation of a registry for human embryonic stem cells carrying an inherited defect: joint collaboration between ESHRE and hESCreg. Hum Reprod. 2009;24(7):1556–60.

Stephenson EL, Mason C, Braude PR. Preimplantation genetic diagnosis as a source of human embryonic stem cells for disease research and drug discovery. BJOG. 2009;116(2):158–65.

Stephenson E, Jacquet L, Miere C, Wood V, Kadeva N, Cornwell G, Codognotto S, Dajani Y, Braude P, Ilic D. Derivation and propagation of human embryonic stem cell lines from frozen embryos in an animal product-free environment. Nat Prot. 2012;7:1366–81.

Strulovici Y, Leopold PL, O'Connor TP, Pergolizzi RG, Crystal RG. Human embryonic stem cells and gene therapy. Mol Ther. 2007;15(5):850–66.

Takahashi K, Tanabe K, Ohnuki M, et al. Induction of pluripotent stem cells from adult human fibroblasts by defined factors. Cell. 2007; 131(5):861–72.

Thomson JA, Itskovitz-Eldor J, Shapiro SS, Waknitz MA, Swiergiel JJ, Marshall VS, Jones JM. Embryonic stem cell lines derived from human blastocysts. Science. 1998;282(5391):1145–7.

Chapter 15
Ethical and Social Aspects of PGD

Clare Williams and Steven Paul Wainwright

The use of PGD is increasing and its indications are expanding, thereby raising important social and ethical questions. Some of these have been raised in earlier chapters but this chapter summarises key work from several distinct disciplinary perspectives – from science and medicine, where the concern is with the *practicalities* of dealing with social and ethical issues; from bioethics, where the focus is often on philosophical analysis that 'pushes the boundaries' of what *should* be done; and from sociology, which draws on social research with patients, scientists and clinicians to offer nuanced accounts of the *complexities* of 'PGD in action'.

C. Williams, BSc, MSc, PhD (✉)
Department of Sociology and Communications,
School of Social Sciences, Brunel University,
Uxbridge, Middlesex UB8 3PH, UK
e-mail: clare.williams@brunel.ac.uk

S.P. Wainwright, BSc, MSc, PhD
Department of Sociology and Communications,
Brunel University London, Middlesex, London, UK
e-mail: steven.wainwright@brunel.ac.uk

T. El-Toukhy, P. Braude (eds.), *Preimplantation Genetic Diagnosis in Clinical Practice*, DOI 10.1007/978-1-4471-2948-6_15,
© Springer-Verlag London 2014

Is PGD Ethically More Acceptable Than PND?

If a couple wish to avoid the birth of a child who would be affected by what they consider to be a serious disability, this is an indication for PGD or for PND followed by termination of pregnancy (TOP). Both techniques are stressful and invasive, and importantly, both involve selection against disability. For those who support the view that life starts at fertilisation and that all forms of human life deserve respect, both procedures involve the intentional creation and subsequent destruction of an embryo. However, proponents of PGD argue that the difference in the timing of the test is significant. First, it is argued that although they should be treated with respect because of their future potential, human embryos before implantation [potential life] are rudimentary in development and thus have a relatively low moral status and limited rights in comparison to a fetus at 12 weeks of gestation [developing life]. Some also argue that discarding embryos based on their genetic potential is not morally different to discarding embryos during IVF treatment based on their likely implantation potential, a process which is widely accepted as part of the assisted conception process. It is also argued that PGD eliminates the anxiety experienced by prospective parents during the first few weeks of spontaneous pregnancy before PND can be performed, even if the pregnancy later proves to be unaffected by the genetic condition.

PGD for Late-Onset and Susceptibility Conditions

Whilst many would support the application of PGD for serious genetic conditions that manifest early in life, it is perhaps more challenging to accept the principle of creating and destroying embryos for the purpose of testing for late-onset conditions such as Huntington or Alzheimer's disease. These conditions allow the affected person around four or five decades of healthy life before symptoms of the disease develop. Furthermore, testing for lower penetrance genes such as cancer predisposition genes often provides a risk assessment, but no definitive information as to whether the condition will develop in later life. It is also feared that selecting for non-medical traits such as intelligence, height, hair, eye colour or athletic genotypes (so-called *designer babies*) will follow.

The use of PGD for late-onset disorders with high penetrance raises concerns in relation to the welfare of any child who might be born to a person with the condition and who is likely to become unwell or even die whilst the child is still dependent on that person for care. This concern is relevant and applies to many similar situations of IVF such as treating an infertile couple where one or both partners are HIV positive or providing gamete or embryo cryopreservation before cancer treatment. However, it is generally accepted that as long as another parent or a competent care provider will be available for the child, the possibility of losing a parent does not justify withholding PGD.

In relation to PGD for lower penetrance genes, most of the UK-based PGD staff interviewed for a study at the time this became possible ultimately felt that parental choice and autonomy should lead the decision-making process. It was acknowledged that having a child with an inherited susceptibility to a disease such as cancer or progressive neurological disorder leading to an early death could be a considerable source of suffering for both child and parents.

The use of PGD to select for non-medical traits has raised many social and ethical questions including whether parental reproductive interests justify creating and destroying human embryos; whether testing for such traits could possibly harm the resulting children, stigmatise existing persons or even create far-reaching social harm by ultimately limiting biodiversity and uniqueness; and what the role of PGD health care professionals should be in relation to decision-making. However, at the current time, screening to select for mental and/or physical desirable characteristics (*the designer baby model*) is unrealistic due to a number of factors including the complex multifactorial genetic nature of these traits, the limited number of embryos created during a PGD cycle and the burdens of undergoing IVF in general.

In a ground-breaking social study of PGD in the UK, Franklin and Roberts explored the views of couples undergoing PGD. In contrast to the notion of 'designer babies' being manufactured for overly fussy parents, they found PGD patients had a 'strong sense of obligation to steer a responsible course away from avoidable harm'. In addition, rather than offering 'unprecedented genetic possibility', PGD was seen by couples themselves as the only alternative, the 'only choice'. In fact, amongst the majority of PGD patients interviewed, the term 'designer baby' was seen as an abusive term and resented by them. As one of the patients interviewed puts it, 'It's not as if we're going to this Unit with a shopping list saying we want this and this. It's more a case of, we're looking for this [genetic disease] because that's what you want to eradicate'.

Franklin and Roberts also argue that the image of PGD as a 'slippery slope' technology which is 'outpacing society's ability to restrict or control its use overlooks the long history of critical assessment and public debate that has surrounded it', with the concerns of those who work in PGD crucially helping to shape the restricted use of the technology, in the UK at least. Further, they believe that this 'demonstrates a serious and concerted attempt to make it as accountable as possible to public scrutiny'.

Fate of Carrier Embryos

In the majority of recessive disorders, carriers remain healthy throughout their lives. However, female carriers of some conditions such as X-linked Duchenne muscular dystrophy may themselves develop some symptoms of the disease. In these cases, selection against carrier embryos may be justified.

The principal motive to select against 'healthy' carrier embryos is to protect the health of the grandchildren rather than the children. The magnitude of the risk to the grandchildren will depend on the mode of inheritance, prevalence and penetrance of the genetic condition. For example, in X-linked disorders, all sons of female carriers will have a 50 % chance of getting the disease, whilst 50 % of daughters will be carriers. Conversely, carriers of a rare autosomal recessive disorder will have a very low risk of facing a difficult reproductive decision unless their partner was also to carry the same rare genetic mutation.

Thus, families undergoing PGD treatment and their physicians are faced with a number of choices. The first is to transfer all 'unaffected' embryos, non-carriers as well as carriers. In support of this policy, it can be argued that carrier embryos are likely to grow into healthy individuals (the prime objective of PGD) and that selecting against carrier embryos stigmatises carriers and could be viewed as a form of positive eugenics. The second choice is not to transfer carrier embryos, in order to prevent future reproductive dilemmas. Although this option may be ethically acceptable to some, with the limited number of embryos suitable for transfer after PGD, it may well lessen the chances of a successful cycle, resulting in the couple undergoing additional PGD cycles, even though there are 'unaffected' carrier embryos available.

Sex Selection for Non-medical Reasons

Identification of the sex of preimplantation embryos in order to avoid X-linked diseases is the third most common indication for PGD after monogenic diseases and chromosomal abnormalities and is generally thought to be ethically acceptable. However, sex selection to serve parental interests in having a child of a particular gender (i.e. social sex selection) is contentious, especially as embryos not of the desired sex are usually discarded. This request may be made either for the first child (where the overwhelming preference internationally is for a male child) or for a second or subsequent children of the opposite sex to the existing one(s) with no greater preference of males over females, so-called family balancing. By definition, social sex selection is not a therapeutic intervention, as it does not prevent a medical harm to any party and confers no advantage to the selected child. Article 14 of the Convention on Human Rights and Biomedicine states that 'the use of techniques of medically assisted procreation shall not be allowed for the purpose of choosing a future's child sex, except when serious hereditary sex-related disease is to be avoided'. This practice is currently prohibited in the UK. Opponents of social sex selection by PGD regard it as immoral and inherently sexist, particularly towards women, because it does not show respect for the 50 % of healthy embryos that are destined to be discarded purely because of their sex. It also sends a strong signal that social sex selection in pregnancy may be legitimate. Some argue that this application of PGD sets a precedent for positive eugenics applications including selection for desirable physical traits for those who can pay for them.

Proponents of social sex selection, on the other hand, view it as an expression of parental reproductive autonomy and argue that PGD is too expensive to be so widely practised as to contribute to sex ratio disparities. It is argued that parents who seek family balancing are unlikely to devalue one or the other sex but simply wish to enjoy the different experiences that come with rearing children of opposite genders. It is also feared that if PGD is not permitted, pregnancy and abortion might be practised instead. Indeed, the Ethics committee of the American Society for Reproductive Medicine concluded in 2001 that sex selection for purposes of variety, but not for the first child, was acceptable, thereby legitimising the desire to raise children of both genders.

Conversely, the Human Fertilisation and Embryology Authority (HFEA) in the UK carried out a public consultation in 2002–2003, which demonstrated a negative public attitude towards PGD for non-medical sex selection. This attitude was also reflected in a more recent study conducted in the north-east of England, which found that 83 % of participants were against the use of prenatal social sex selection.

PGD for HLA-Typing

PGD has been used to enable families to have a child who is a tissue match for an existing sick sibling in need of an allogeneic haematopoietic stem cell (HSC) transplant because of bone marrow disorders including leukaemia, Diamond-Blackfan anaemia (DBA), Fanconi anaemia, β-thalassemia major and severe combined immunodeficiency syndrome (SCID). The success of the transplant depends largely on the HLA match between the donor and recipient. In many situations the sooner the HSC transplant is performed, the greater its success rate will be.

PGD can be performed to ensure that only those embryos that are a tissue match (about 25 % of all embryos) are transferred to the woman. However, it should be remembered that leukaemia and DBA in the sibling are often sporadic and the matched embryos (future children) are not at risk of developing the same disease. Critics argue against this use of PGD, stating that an embryo (and the child it will become) should not be exposed to the risks of PGD, unless that embryo/person is likely to derive enough benefit to outweigh these risks. The complexity of the debate increases significantly when considering the limits that should be placed on what the donor child should undergo in order to treat a sick sibling. For example, collecting umbilical cord blood at birth is non-invasive and thus widely seen as acceptable, whilst harvesting bone marrow stem cells or vital organs such as a kidney from the HLA-matched child constitutes a much more difficult social and ethical situation in view of the risks involved for the donor child. It is also argued that a child should be created, raised and valued in its own right and should not to be used instrumentally as a means to an end (to serve as a donor for the existing sick sibling).

On the other hand, those who support its use argue that parents have children for many instrumental reasons including to save a marriage, continuity of the family, as well as for economic and psychological benefits to parents. Importantly, this is not considered unethical as long as the child is also valued in its own right, since people are judged on their attitudes towards children rather than on their motives for having them. The fact that these parents make so much physical, emotional and often financial effort to save their sick child suggests that they are responsible, loving parents and that children conceived in order to save an existing child are likely to be loved and valued for their own sake as well as for the added benefit they confer by potentially saving the sick sibling. As PGD is not an easy or guaranteed solution for the family involved, decisions about such complex cases are generally made on a case-by-case basis, after weighing up carefully the potential risks and benefits to all those involved.

PGD and Stem Cell Science

Scientists have argued that PGD embryos with an 'unclear diagnosis' cannot be implanted and that these 'spare embryos' form an ethical source for the development of embryonic stem cell lines. Some of the first human embryonic stem cell lines in the UK came from such PGD embryos. More recently, embryos affected with a genetic disease have been used to develop so-called 'disease-in-a-dish' models. Proponents argue that these human cell lines enable scientists to understand the genetic nature of many diseases that currently have poor or no treatment and these new models of disease could offer hope for the development of potent, novel drugs.

Conclusion

PGD offers the technological promise of increased reproductive choice and a new era of *predictive medicine*. However, the application of PGD is replete with social and ethical problems, and it can be envisaged that increasingly complicated cases will continue to present themselves in the future as new technologies emerge. It is the social and moral duty of society to debate the implications inherent to the use of PGD for various indications. More work addressing the safety, reliability and effectiveness of PGD is also needed to enhance this process.

Key Points
- The uses of PGD are expanding as are its social and ethical implications.
- PGD for late-onset and susceptibility conditions requires careful consideration on a case-by-case basis.
- PGD for gender selection for non-medical reasons is prohibited in the UK.
- PGD embryos are an important source of embryonic stem cells and for producing human disease models for the development of new drugs.

Further Reading

El-Toukhy T, Williams C, Braude P. The ethics of PGD. Obstet Gynaecol. 2008;10:49–54.

Franklin S, Roberts C. Born and made: an ethnography of preimplantation genetic diagnosis. Pittsburgh: Pittsburgh University Press; 2006.

Scully JL, Banks S, Shakespeare TW. Chance, choice and control: lay debate on prenatal social sex selection. Soc Sci Med. 2006;63:21–31.

Wainwright SP, Michael M, Williams C. Shifting paradigms? Reflections on regenerative medicine, embryonic stem cells and pharmaceuticals. Sociol Health Illn. 2008;30:959–74.

Williams C, Ehrich K, Farsides B, Scott R. Facilitating choice, framing choice: staff views on widening the scope of PGD in the UK. Soc Sci Med. 2007;65:1094–105.

Williams C, Wainwright SP, Ehrich K, Michael M. Human embryos as boundary objects? Some reflections on the biomedical worlds of embryonic stem cells and pre-implantation genetic diagnosis. New Genet Soc. 2008;27:7–8.

Chapter 16
Preimplantation Genetic Screening

Sjoerd Repping, Sebastiaan Mastenbroek, and Paul N. Scriven

Embryo Selection by the Use of PGS

In the majority of in vitro fertilization (IVF) cycles, multiple embryos are created after ovarian stimulation. The viability of these embryos, and, as a consequence, the chances of an embryo implanting successfully, is subject to biological variation. To achieve the best possible live birth rates after IVF while minimizing the risk for multiple pregnancy, one or two embryos considered to have the best chances of implanting are selected for transfer. Subsequently, supernumerary good quality embryos are selected for cryopreservation and possible

S. Repping, PhD • S. Mastenbroek, PhD (✉)
Center for Reproductive Medicine, Academic Medical Center,
University of Amsterdam, Meibergdreef 9,
Amsterdam, 1105 AZ, The Netherlands
e-mail: s.repping@amc.nl; s.mastenbroek@amc.nl

P.N. Scriven, BSc, PhD
Medical & Molecular Genetics, King's College London Medical
School, Cytogenetics, 5th Floor Tower Wing, Guy's Hospital,
Great Maze Pond, London SE1 9RT, UK
e-mail: paul.scriven@kcl.ac.uk

T. El-Toukhy, P. Braude (eds.), *Preimplantation Genetic
Diagnosis in Clinical Practice*, DOI 10.1007/978-1-4471-2948-6_16,
© Springer-Verlag London 2014

transfer in the future, while remaining embryos of poor quality with little or no implantation potential are discarded.

Since the earliest days of IVF, the method of choice for embryo selection has been morphological evaluation, but with this type of embryo selection, implantation rates in general do not exceed 35 %. This has resulted in a strong drive to find alternative selection methods.

Based on the high incidence of numerical chromosomal abnormalities found in preimplantation embryos, preimplantation genetic screening (PGS) has been proposed as a method to select embryos for transfer in an IVF treatment. In PGS, typically a single blastomere is biopsied from each embryo, and the copy number of a set of chromosomes is then determined in that blastomere. Subsequently, embryos that are identified as abnormal (aneuploidy) are discarded, and embryos with a normal genetic constitution (euploid) are selected for transfer.

The Genetic Constitution of Human Embryos

The human haploid chromosome number (n) is 23, one copy of each autosome (numbered 1–22) and either the X or Y chromosome (Chap. 2). A euploid chromosome complement is a multiple of the haploid chromosome number. Following female and male meiosis, a haploid oocyte and spermatozoon fuse and become a diploid ($2n$) zygote with 46 chromosomes, 22 pairs of autosomes and an XX (female) or XY (male) sex chromosome pair. An aneuploid chromosome complement is any numerical deviation from euploidy and includes chromosome loss or gain. This can arise due to malsegregation of chromosomes during meiosis or during post-zygotic mitotic cell division. For a diploid complement, the gain or loss of a single chromosome results in trisomy (three copies) or monosomy (one copy) and chromosome imbalance.

In general chromosome imbalance is incompatible with life. Monosomy is almost always lethal at an early stage and is rarely found in a recognizable pregnancy. Trisomy is usually lethal before birth but in some cases can be viable, trisomy 13, 18 and 21, causing Patau, Edwards and Down syndrome, respectively. Although viable, these individuals have profound mental and physical disability. Trisomy 21 has the greatest potential to be viable, although fewer than 1 in 5 conceptions reach term and only 1 in 50 in trisomy 13 conceptions.

In most cases chromosome aneuploidy is sporadic; however, the incidence increases with maternal age; for example, the incidence of trisomy 21 is 1 in 1,440 when a woman is 20 years of age and 1 in 84 when she is 40. In clinically recognized pregnancies, aneuploidies occur more frequently when a woman is over 35 years old. At the same time, it is in these women that pregnancy chances decline sharply both in normal conception and after IVF.

Herein lies the rationale for PGS: excluding from transfer embryos with an abnormal chromosome complement should result in an increase in live birth rates after IVF. In addition, the transfer of embryos with a normal genetic constitution should reduce the chance of a miscarriage.

The Technology of PGS

A sample for genetic testing can be obtained from the oocyte preconception (the first polar body only) or postconception from the zygote (the second polar body), from the cleavage-stage embryo (1 or 2 day 3 blastomeres) or from a day 5 or 6 blastocyst (several trophectoderm cells). A limitation of testing polar bodies is that it can only identify aneuploidy of maternal origin. Testing blastomeres has the advantage that meiotic aneuploidy originating from either parent can be detected. However, errors in mitotic cell division in the early embryo can result in cells with different chromosome complements (mosaicism) in the same embryo; these can be different combinations of aneuploid cells or a mixture of diploid and aneuploid cells. This is important

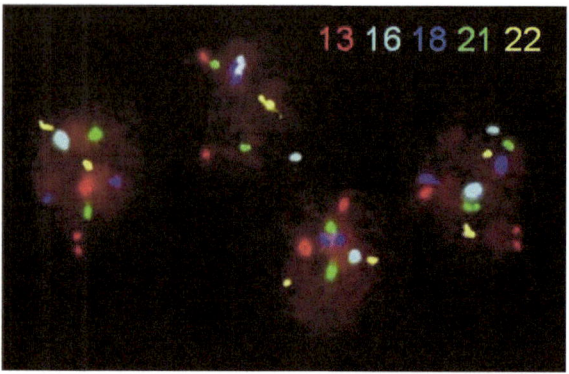

FIGURE. 16.1 Interphase nuclei hybridized with FISH probes specific for sequences on chromosomes 13, 16, 18, 21 and 22, two signals of the same colour indicate normal copy number, one signal monosomy and three signals trisomy

because the diagnostic accuracy of an aneuploidy test using any technology depends on the sample being representative of the embryo. It is important to appreciate that the predictive value of an abnormal result following indiscriminate testing of embryos where the incidence of aneuploidy might be low, even in the best hands, risks being no better than tossing a coin.

Since the introduction of PGS in 1995, the primary technique to identify chromosome aneuploidy in a single cell has been fluorescence in situ hybridization (FISH). Chromosome-specific sequences of DNA tagged with fluorophores of different colours (DNA probes) can be used to count the number of chromosomes present in a polar body or the nucleus of a blastomere or trophectoderm cell and differentiate a diploid chromosome complement from other euploid complements [haploid (1n), triploid (3n) and tetraploid (4n)] and aneuploid complements with monosomy and/ or trisomy for one or more individual chromosomes tested. The FISH technique is limited by there being relatively few discrete colours available and typically up to five chromosomes can be tested at the same time (Fig. 16.1). However,

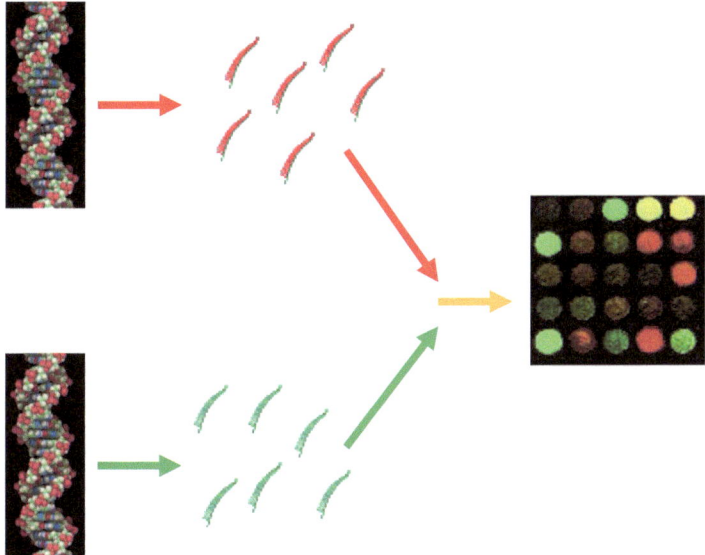

FIGURE. 16.2 Cartoon representation of principle of array CGH. Total genomic DNA from test material is prepared as small fragments and labelled with a red fluorochrome, then mixed with reference DNA similarly prepared and labelled with a green fluorochrome. The mixed pool of DNA is added to the array slide, where sequences compete for complementary sequences on the slide. The resulting fluorescence ratios give information on the relative copy number of each sequence

the same nucleus can be retested (reprobed) and in this way 12 chromosomes have been tested in clinical practice. High technical skill is required, and scoring FISH signals in a single nucleus is inherently subjective and prone to errors.

More recent application of microarray technology to PGS has made it possible to test for aneuploidy for every chromosome. Array CGH is a technique where whole-genome amplified DNA from the biopsied sample and a normal reference sample is labelled with different fluorophores (red and green) and hybridized to thousands of specific DNA segments of known size and location from every chromosome located on a glass slide (Fig. 16.2). Although capable of detecting all chromosomes, and their loss or gain, a disadvantage of this technique is that it cannot differentiate quantitatively between a normal diploid-euploid complement (e.g. 46,XX) and abnormal euploid complements (e.g. haploid 23,X; triploid 69,XXX; tetraploid 92,XXXX). Although relatively rare at conception, triploidy is found in 16 % of spontaneous miscarriages.

A different microarray technique exploits the common occurrence (around ten million have been identified) of single nucleotide polymorphisms (SNP) throughout the genome. These are DNA sequences where there is a single nucleotide difference between a pair of chromosomes at the same location (e.g. GATTACA and GATTTCA) and therefore heterozygous alleles. SNP arrays typically use hundreds of thousands of probes (high-density arrays). An advantage of SNP array analysis is that the copy number of each chromosome present can be independently verified using the degree of allele heterozygosity. Where only one copy of a chromosome is present (single copy loss, monosomy), there is only one SNP allele at every locus and there is loss of heterozygosity. Where there are three copies of a chromosome (single copy gain, trisomy), the number of alleles is increased at every locus on the chromosome.

How Does PGS Differ from PGD?

A distinction between PGS and PGD is not universally recognized. In contrast to PGD, PGS is primarily associated with attempting to improve the efficiency of ART, whereas the primary objective of PGD is to give disadvantaged couples with serious inherited genetic conditions the same chance of a healthy child as any couple in the general population. For PGD the pregnancy rate may be of secondary concern to the increased risks of having a child affected with a serious genetic disorder or having the difficult decision to terminate an affected pregnancy. Advanced technologies currently available seek to combine testing for inherited genetic conditions (i.e. PGD) with sporadic chromosome aneuploidy (i.e. PGS). Whether this holds any clinical benefit for the couple undergoing PGD has not been fully explored.

The 'Indication' for PGS

Given the aforementioned correlation between maternal age and the decreased chance of pregnancy as well as the increased incidence of aneuploidy, the beneficial effect of PGS was expected to be greatest in women of advanced maternal age. Next to women of advanced maternal age, PGS has been offered to women with a history of recurrent miscarriage, women with a history of repeated implantation failure (i.e. several failed IVF cycles) and women whose partner has poor sperm quality (severe male factor), mainly because of the high incidence of aneuploidy detected in the embryos of these women. More recently, PGS has also been offered to younger women (under 35 years of age), as high aneuploidy rates were also found in their embryos.

What Is the Evidence?

In 1995, the first deliveries were reported after transfer of embryos that had been screened for aneuploidies. Since then the use of PGS has become increasingly common, in particular among women considered to be of advanced maternal age. Some have even suggested that PGS should become a standard procedure for all women undergoing IVF.

Observational studies comparing IVF with and without PGS carried out in the 1990s and the early years of this century demonstrated that PGS is associated with higher implantation rates per transferred embryo, but not with an increase in the rate of ongoing pregnancies per initiated cycle or per oocyte retrieval.

Rigorous scientific evidence on the effectiveness of PGS has only come in recent years. Nine randomized controlled trials comparing IVF with and without PGS have thus far been conducted. FISH was used in all trials and cleavage-stage biopsy was used in all but one. PGS significantly lowered live birth rate after IVF for women of advanced maternal age (risk difference −0.08, 95 %; CI −0.13 to −0.03); for a live birth rate of 26 % after IVF without PGS, the rate would be between 13 and 23 % using PGS. Trials where PGS was offered to women with a good prognosis and to women with repeated implantation failure suggested similar outcomes.

Thus, currently there is no evidence of a beneficial effect of PGS on the live birth rate after IVF using cleavage-stage biopsy and FISH. On the contrary, for women of advanced maternal age, PGS significantly lowers the live birth rate. Likewise, there is no rigorous scientific evidence on the efficacy of the more recently developed PGS methods.

The reason behind the inability of PGS to increase live birth rates lies in part in the technology itself and in part in the biology of the human preimplantation embryo. Technically, PGS could negatively affect embryo development because it requires the removal of one or two blastomeres at the cleavage stage. In addition, the molecular techniques used to determine chromosome copy number are not flawless (see Chap. 6). Biologically, the high incidence of chromosomal mosaicism at the cleavage stage undermines the principle that the cell analyzed in PGS resembles the entire embryo. Cumulative data from the literature suggests that over half of all day 3 human preimplantation embryos are diploid-aneuploid mosaic.

Is Selection the Way Forward?

The widespread use and recent development and optimization of PGS is driven by the concept that better embryo selection will improve the success rates of IVF, since embryos that are cryopreserved have a reduced chance of implanting after thawing. Better selection methods should result in higher live birth rates without an increase in multiple pregnancies.

Recent developments challenge this concept and suggest that perhaps the path of embryo selection is turning into a dead end in the quest for optimal IVF success rates. The main reason is the accumulating evidence that all embryos can now be cryopreserved and transferred in subsequent cycles without significantly impairing pregnancy rates or perhaps even with better pregnancy rates. Furthermore, recent data suggest that babies that result from such freeze/thaw cycles are healthier than babies that result from fresh transfer of embryos. No selection method will ever lead to improved live birth rates in a 'freeze-all scenario', as, by definition, the live birth rate per stimulated IVF cycle can never be improved upon when all embryos are serially transferred. In fact, if the selection method under study would not be 100 % specific, then selection would even lower the live birth rate after IVF, as some viable embryos are incorrectly discarded instead of being transferred. The only parameter that could possibly be improved upon by embryo selection would be time to pregnancy, provided embryos with the highest implantation potential are transferred first. At present, there is no one PGS method that has been proven to be 100 % specific.

A Future for PGS

The inefficacy of PGS using cleavage-stage biopsy and FISH has in recent years led to a renewed and increasing interest in further development of, and adjustments to, the PGS technique. New methods to determine the ploidy status of a single cell, such as microarrays, are being studied. In an attempt to avoid the confounding effects of chromosomal mosaicism, embryos are now biopsied at either the zygote or blastocyst stage. Despite the complete lack of rigorous evidence of benefit of these new methods, many have already been implemented into clinical practice at least in some clinics. Indeed, the theory behind these developments sounds plausible, the techniques used are attractive and provide potential and the first results seem promising. However, a decade ago, this was exactly the scenario when PGS using cleavage-stage biopsy and FISH was promoted and introduced into clinical practice.

It is important that prior to wholesale implementation, practitioners first provide robust evidence of method assessment and controlled pilot studies to allow rigorous clinical trials on the efficacy of new PGS techniques to be conducted. In the event of future studies indeed showing that all embryos of an IVF cycle can be cryopreserved and transferred in subsequent cycles without impairing pregnancy rates (or maybe even with an improvement in pregnancy rates), then such RCTs of PGS are of limited value, as no form of PGS will ever improve the live birth rate after IVF in such a scenario. It will only be able to potentially decrease time to pregnancy.

Key Points
- Chromosome aneuploidy is naturally occurring, typically sporadic and generally leads to non-viable offspring.
- PGS has the potential to select the best embryos for transfer and reduce the risk of losing a much wanted pregnancy.
- There is no high-level clinical evidence from randomized control trials of a beneficial effect of PGS on the live birth rate after IVF.
- For women of advanced age, PGS using cleavage-stage biopsy and FISH leads to a significant decrease in live birth rates.
- Technical limitations and chromosomal mosaicism confound the effectiveness of PGS. A test that identifies aneuploidy with 100 % accuracy would be a significant advance; however, such a test has not yet been developed.
- New approaches in the application of PGS should be evaluated carefully before their introduction into clinical practice.
- Further development of the so-called freeze-all strategies would make any selection method, including PGS, of limited value.

Further Reading

Aflatoonian A, Oskouian H, Ahmadi S, Oskouian L. Can fresh embryo transfers be replaced by cryopreserved-thawed embryo transfers in assisted reproductive cycles? A randomized controlled trial. J Assist Reprod Genet. 2010;27:357–63.

Baart EB, Martini E, van den Berg I, Macklon NS, Galjaard RJ, Fauser BC, Van Opstal D. Preimplantation genetic screening reveals a high incidence of aneuploidy and mosaicism in embryos from young women undergoing IVF. Hum Reprod. 2006;21:223–33.

Bisignano A, Wells D, Harton G, Munné S. PGD and aneuploidy screening for 24 chromosomes: advantages and disadvantages of competing platforms. Reprod Biomed Online. 2011;23:677–85.

Centers for Disease Control and Prevention, American Society for Reproductive Medicine, and Society for Assisted Reproductive Technology (2010) 2008 Assisted reproductive technology success rates: national summary and fertility clinic reports. http://apps.nccd. cdc.gov/art/Apps/NationalSummaryReport.aspx

Gardner RJM, Sutherland GR, Shaffer LG. Chromosome abnormalities and genetic counseling. 4th ed. New York: Oxford University Press; 2012.

Gleicher N, Barad DH. A review of, and commentary on, the ongoing second clinical introduction of preimplantation genetic screening (PGS) to routine IVF practice. J Assist Reprod Genet. 2012;29(11): 1159–66.

Hassold T, Hunt P. To err (meiotically) is human: the genesis of human aneuploidy. Nat Rev Genet. 2001;2:280–91.

Mastenbroek S, Twisk M, van der Veen F, Repping S. Preimplantation genetic screening: a systematic review and meta-analysis of RCTs. Hum Reprod Update. 2011;17:454–66.

Mastenbroek S, van der Veen F, Aflatoonian A, Shapiro B, Bossuyt P, Repping S. Embryo selection in IVF. Hum Reprod. 2011;26:964–6.

Munné S, Wells D, Cohen J. Technology requirements for preimplantation genetic diagnosis to improve assisted reproduction outcomes. Fertil Steril. 2010;94:408–30.

Nagy ZP. Symposium: innovative techniques in human embryo viability assessment. Reprod Biomed Online. 2008;17:451–507.

Scriven PN, Ogilvie CM, Khalaf Y. Embryo selection in IVF: is polar body array comparative genomic hybridization accurate enough? Hum Reprod. 2012;27:951–3.

van Echten-Arends J, Mastenbroek S, Sikkema-Raddatz B, et al. Chromosomal mosaicism in human preimplantation embryos: a systematic review. Hum Reprod Update. 2011;17(5):620–7.

Verlinsky Y, Cohen J, Munne S, Gianaroli L, Simpson JL, Ferraretti AP, Kuliev A. Over a decade of experience with preimplantation genetic diagnosis: a multicenter report. Fertil Steril. 2004;82:292–4.

Chapter 17
Regulation of PGD in the UK and Worldwide

Veronica English and Peter Braude

Assisted reproduction, including preimplantation genetic diagnosis, has been subject to statutory regulation in the UK since 1991. The Human Fertilisation and Embryology Act (1990) based largely on the recommendations of the 1984 Inquiry into Human Fertilisation and Embryology (the Warnock Report) made it a criminal offence to carry out certain activities without a licence from the statutory regulatory body, the Human Fertilisation and Embryology Authority (HFEA). The activities that required a licence were:

- The creation or use of human embryos in vitro, for treatment or research (including preimplantation genetic diagnosis)
- The use of donated gametes or embryos
- The storage of gametes and embryos

V. English, BA (Hons) (✉)
Department of Medical Ethics, British Medical Association,
BMA House, Tavistock Square, London WC1H 9JP, UK
e-mail: venglish@bma.org.uk

P. Braude, MB, BCh, PhD, FRCOG, FMedSci, FSB
Division of Women's Health, King's College London,
St. Thomas' Hospital, Westminster Bridge Road,
London SE1 7EH, UK
e-mail: peter.braude@kcl.ac.uk

T. El-Toukhy, P. Braude (eds.), *Preimplantation Genetic Diagnosis in Clinical Practice*, DOI 10.1007/978-1-4471-2948-6_17, © Springer-Verlag London 2014

This list was extended in 2007 to include some other forms of fertility treatment and clinical procedures in order to comply with the EU Tissues and Cells Directive.

Regulating PGD Under the 1990 Act

The first successful application of PGD in two couples happened whilst Parliament was debating the 1990 Act. Although aware of the potential use of PGD for avoiding disability, it chose not to set out detailed criteria for its use in the Act. Instead it gave the HFEA the power to issue treatment licences to authorise, in the course of providing treatment services, 'practices designed to secure that embryos are in a suitable condition to be placed in a woman or to determine whether embryos are suitable for that purpose'. This placed sole responsibility for setting the boundaries within which PGD could take place firmly within the remit of the HFEA, until Parliament revisited the issue in 2008 (see below). Consistent with the 'special status' of the embryo reflected in both the Warnock Report and the legislation, the HFEA decided at an early stage that embryo testing should be restricted to cases where a child would be at significant risk of serious harm – albeit the word 'serious' was not defined. This made the criteria for testing and the disposal of affected embryos consistent with the legal criteria, in the Abortion Act 1967 (as amended), for termination of an existing pregnancy on grounds of fetal abnormality. In line with this position, the HFEA also made clear that although the use of PGD to determine the sex of embryos in order to avoid serious X-linked conditions was permitted, the technique must not be used to select the sex of a child for social reasons.

Assessing Technical Proficiency

Any clinic undertaking PGD in the UK must be licensed by the HFEA to perform IVF treatment and meet all of the criteria set out in the HFEA's code of practice. In addition, between

1999 and 2009, individual embryo biopsy practitioners were required to apply to the HFEA to be 'registered' to carry out the procedure. In order to achieve this status, they had to provide evidence of their competence and expertise, from the use of embryos donated for research, and to be inspected and assessed by an HFEA inspector. Only those practitioners registered with the HFEA for this purpose could undertake embryo biopsy procedures in clinical practice. The responsibility for ensuring the competence of embryo biopsy practitioners now falls to the 'Person Responsible' (who under the Act is the individual legally responsible for the practice in the clinic) who must ensure that their performance is regularly assessed.

Conditions For Which PGD May Be Used

The HFEA has always rejected the idea of producing a list of medical conditions that it considers sufficiently serious to justify the use of PGD. Rather each individual condition is considered as and when an application for its use is received. By law, each condition for which PGD is intended must be approved as appropriate by the HFEA before PGD may take place. Initially, individual clinics were required to apply for a licence for each condition for which it wished to test, but since October 2009, once a condition has been approved by the HFEA in principle, any clinic in the UK licensed to practice PGD was able to test for that condition without the need to submit its own separate application. A list of approved conditions is provided on the HFEA's website.

Assessing Seriousness

The issue of 'seriousness' was addressed in a public consultation exercise undertaken by the HFEA in 1999. Whilst determined to maintain its approach of ensuring consistency with prenatal diagnosis, the Authority wanted to explore some of the boundaries and provide some general guidance about how seriousness should be assessed in this context. Much debate focused on whether there should be some form of objective test of seriousness or whether it was appropriate to take into account the experiences and perspectives of the individuals concerned. The HFEA concluded that the family's own perspective of the seriousness of the disease *for them*, given their individual circumstances, was an important factor to take into account. This general principle guides both the HFEA's decision making about individual conditions and the decisions of individual clinics about whether to provide PGD in a particular case. In its code of practice (HFEA 2009), the HFEA advises clinics to consider:

- The views of the people seeking treatment in relation to the condition to be avoided, including their previous reproductive experience
- The likely degree of suffering association with the condition
- The availability of effective therapy now and in the future
- The speed of degeneration in progressive disorders
- The extent of any intellectual impairment
- The social support available
- The family circumstances of the people seeking treatment

Assessing 'Significant Risk'

In the early days of PGD, the conditions tested for were congenital or childhood-onset conditions with near full penetrance. In all such cases there would be a 'significant risk' that a child born would suffer from the disorder. As our knowledge and understanding of genetics increased, however, the question arose as to how immediate or likely the risk had to be to be considered 'significant'. The first challenge was a request for the use of PGD for Huntington's disease, a serious disorder which does not manifest until well into adulthood – a late onset disorder (see Chaps. 3 and 4). Whilst the baby and later the child would not be at 'significant' risk of the disorder, the adult he or she grew into would be. Another challenge to the significance test arose in relation to testing embryos for conditions with a far lower penetrance, such as some forms of cancer where those with the mutation are at a 30–80 % lifetime risk of developing the condition. In such cases, the child or later adult, derived from an 'affected' embryo, may never develop the condition. In some cases, such as inherited forms of breast cancer, the condition would be both late onset, with the possibility of screening or treatment available, and of lower penetrance (discussed in Chap. 4).

The HFEA once again set out to gauge public and professional opinion before ruling on such cases (HFEA 2005). Guided by this consultation exercise, and the views of its own Ethics and Law Committee, it concluded that, in principle, it was appropriate that PGD should be available for serious, lower penetrance, later-onset genetic conditions such as inherited breast, bowel and ovarian cancer. Initially it required each request to be considered by the Authority on a case-by-case basis but this requirement was removed in 2010 when approval for lower penetrance disorders was brought into line with the main PGD licensing system.

Who Is 'the Child' at Risk?

The HFEA's aim for consistency with prenatal diagnosis, with its requirement that *the child* is at significant risk of serious harm, came under further challenge by requests for the use of PGD combined with HLA testing to produce a child who would be a compatible cord blood or tissue donor for a very sick sibling (see Chap. 13). In some of these cases, the child to be born itself was at risk of the condition and so the criteria for PGD were met. However, additional testing was requested to ensure that, of the unaffected embryos, preference should be given to those that would result in a compatible donor for a sibling. In other cases the child to be born was not at risk at all, but was tested solely to ensure compatibility. This not only challenged the HFEA's desire for consistency with prenatal diagnosis but also the legal obligation of all clinics to take account of the 'welfare of any child who may be born or affected by the treatment'. After much deliberation the HFEA concluded that, in principle, it was willing to accept PGD with HLA testing, but initially restricted such testing to cases where the child itself was at risk. This distinction was subsequently removed. Whilst the welfare of the child provisions of the legislation were satisfied by the fact that the treatment was of benefit to another child 'affected by the treatment', in this case, the HEEA had to set to one side its adherence to the principle of consistency with prenatal diagnosis.

Parliamentary Review

In 2008 Parliament had the opportunity to scrutinise the way in which the HFEA had managed the responsibilities delegated to it in respect of PGD. The decisions made by the Authority in the intervening years, and the framework for decision making that had been established, were subsequently endorsed and integrated into the legislation. In place of the general statement about ensuring embryos were suitable for transfer came a new detailed section explicitly addressing PGD. In line with the HFEA's rulings, sex selection other than for medical reasons is prohibited, PGD with HLA testing is permitted and the HFEA can approve testing where there is a risk that the child would have or develop a serious disability, illness or medical condition. The legislation also specifically prohibits the deliberate selection for the purpose of replacement of affected embryos. This follows publicity given to a case in the USA where a deaf couple wanted to use PGD to select a deaf child.

Regulation in Other Countries

The USA does not have federal law that specifically dictates how PGD may be practised and which diseases are or are not suitable for this purpose. The regulatory framework is largely by professional self-regulation or by legislation in individual states. The American Society of Reproductive Medicine issues practice guidelines and, unlike the UK and many other countries in Europe, condones sex selection for non-medical purposes – 'family balancing' (see Chap. 15). The use of PGS thrives there with a number of companies established to provide testing services for multiple conditions using sophisticated molecular techniques (see Chap. 19).

Because individual states in Europe have diverse albeit linked histories, and varying degrees of religious influence, laws about PGD are not unified. In France PGD is regulated by a law that allows healthy embryos to be selected when a parent or other close relative has a serious genetic disease and PGD to provide a tissue match for an ill sibling is also allowed. Sex selection is legal for medical purposes, but not for cultural reasons or family balancing. Italy's Law on Assisted Reproduction 2001 only allows ART for infertile heterosexual couples and also makes it illegal to freeze or destroy human embryos. This was in 2007 successfully challenged in 2007 over a landmark case of PGD for thalassaemia and again in 2012 by the European Court of Human Rights over a PGD case for cystic fibrosis which is being appealed by the Italian government.

In Austria and Germany, neither PGD nor PND was allowed for the purposes of selecting against embryos that may be considered to carry disabling disorders (embryopathic indications). Germany's Embryo Protection Act protects a fertilised egg from the time of fusion of pronuclei and made it a criminal offence to use embryos in a way that does not promote their survival, thus precluding biopsy and PGD. The recent change by free vote (2011) following a landmark case now allows PGD in restricted centres if the chances of a miscarriage or stillbirth are high for genetic reasons or if the parents have strong likelihood of passing on a genetic defect.

Key Points
- It is a criminal offence in the UK to carry out PGD without a licence from the Human Fertilisation and Embryology Authority.
- The HFEA must approve each condition before it is used for the first time in PGD; once approved, other clinics licensed to offer PGD may test for the same condition without seeking approval.
- In most cases, the HFEA will only approve conditions where there is a risk that a child would have or develop a serious disability, illness or medical condition; this could include adult-onset disorders and predisposition to serious conditions.
- The exception to this general rule is PGD with HLA testing in order to select a suitable donor for a very sick sibling, which the HFEA will consider.
- It is unlawful to use PGD to select the sex of a child for social reasons or for the deliberate selection and replacement of affected embryos.
- The law in the rest Europe is varied but changing in favour of allowing PGD. In general sex selection for non-medical purposes is outlawed, unlike the USA where gender selection for family balancing is allowed.

Further Reading

Den Exter A. Embryonic screening as a European Human Right. J Family Reprod Health Care. 2012;6(4). Accessed at: jfrh.tums.ac.ir/index.php/jfrh/article/download/317/313.

HMSO. Report of the committee of inquiry into human fertilisation and embryology (Warnock report) 1984. Accessible at: http://www.hfea.gov.uk/2068.html.

Human Fertilisation and Embryology Authority. Human fertilisation and embryology authority report: preimplantation tissue typing. London: HFEA; 2004.

Human Fertilisation and Embryology Authority. Choices and boundaries. London: HFEA; 2005.

Human Fertilisation and Embryology Authority. Choices and boundaries report. A summary of responses to the HFEA public discussion. London: HFEA; 2006.

Human Fertilisation and Embryology Authority. Authority decision on the use of PGD for lower penetrance, later onset inherited conditions. London: HFEA; 2006.

Human Fertilisation and Embryology Authority. Code of practice. 8th ed. London: HFEA; 2009.

Human Fertilisation and Embryology Authority and Advisory Committee on Genetic Testing. Consultation document on preimplantation genetic diagnosis. London: HFEA; 1999.

Human Fertilisation and Embryology Authority, Human Genetics Commission. Outcome of the public consultation on preimplantation genetic diagnosis. London: HFEA; 2001.

Isasi RM, Knoppers BM. National regulatory frameworks regarding human reproductive genetic testing (preimplantation genetic diagnosis/prenatal diagnosis) a report for the genetics and public policy center. 2006. http://www.dnapolicy.org/pdf/geneticTesting.pdf.

Tuffs A. Germany allows restricted access to preimplantation genetic testing. BMJ. 2011;343:d4425 (Published 12 July 2011).

Turone F. Italian court upholds couple's demand for preimplantation genetic diagnosis. BMJ. 2007;335:687.

Chapter 18
New Developments in PGD

Alison Jones, Pamela Renwick, Alison Lashwood, and Tarek El-Toukhy

PGD is a fast-changing landscape of reproductive medicine and constantly adopts new developments to improve its availability, accuracy and safety. These developments have been made possible because of rapid advances in assisted conception techniques and genetic testing tools. This chapter will

A. Jones, BSc (Hons), MMedSci (✉)
Assisted Conception Unit, Guy's Hospital,
11th Floor, Tower Wing, Great Maze Pond,
London SE1 9RT, UK
e-mail: alison.x.jones@gstt.nhs.uk

P. Renwick, FCRPath, PhD, MSc, BSc
Centre for Preimplantation Genetic Diagnosis,
Guy's and St. Thomas' Hospital, Great Maze Pond,
London SE1 9RT, UK
e-mail: pamela.renwick@gstt.nhs.uk

T. El-Toukhy, MBBCh, MSc, MD, MRCOG
Assisted Conception Unit and PGD Centre, Guy's and St. Thomas'
Hospital NHS Foundation Trust, 11th Floor, Tower Wing,
Guy's Hospital, Great Maze Pond, London SE1 9RT, UK
e-mail: tarek.el-toukhy@gstt.nhs.uk

A. Lashwood, Msc, RGN, RSCN, Dip HV
Clinical Genetics Department, Guy's and St. Thomas' Hospital
NHS Foundation Trust, 7th Floor Borough Wing,
Great Maze Pond, London SE1 9RT, UK
e-mail: alison.lashwood@gstt.nhs.uk

T. El-Toukhy, P. Braude (eds.), *Preimplantation Genetic Diagnosis in Clinical Practice*, DOI 10.1007/978-1-4471-2948-6_18, © Springer-Verlag London 2014

cover some of those new developments, which are gradually being incorporated into the day-to-day PGD service.

With the introduction of new technologies into routine clinical practice, it is imperative that our focus remains on the safety of children born after PGD. Therefore, this chapter will also provide an up-to-date summary of the available literature on the follow-up of PGD babies and children and recommendations for future follow-up studies.

Trophectoderm Biopsy for PGD

Embryo biopsy for PGD is usually performed on day 3 after fertilisation when the embryo has developed to the 6–8 cell stage. One or two cells are removed for testing following breaching of the zona pellucida with acidified Tyrode's solution or a laser. This equates to up to 25 % of the total cell mass of the embryo. Although good results are achieved with cleavage stage biopsy, the biopsy procedure may risk the removal of critical cell mass from the embryo. Many IVF laboratories are routinely culturing embryos to the blastocyst stage using sequential medium and low-oxygen culture systems. This expertise has lead to advances in embryo biopsy techniques with the development of trophectoderm biopsy on day 5 or 6. Trophectoderm biopsy at the blastocyst stage enables many more cells to be removed whilst avoiding damage to the inner cell mass.

Methodology

- Embryos are hatched using a laser on day 3 to encourage herniation of the trophectoderm at the blastocyst stage (Fig. 18.1).
- Early on the morning of day 5, embryos are examined for protruding trophectoderm. If this has not occurred, they are re-examined up to 24 h later.

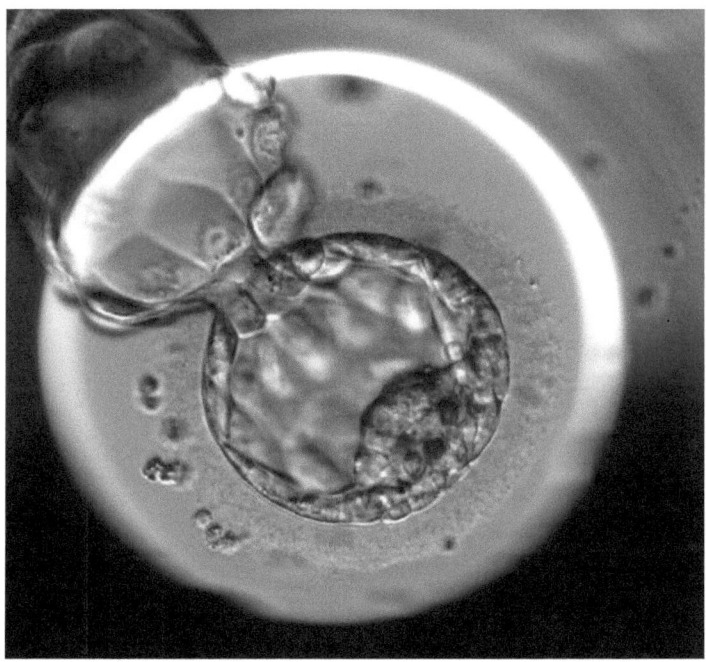

FIGURE 18.1 Herniating blastocyst before trophectoderm biopsy

- Embryos for biopsy are held on a holding pipette with the trophectoderm at the 3 o'clock position. Approximately 5–10 cells are then drawn into a biopsy pipette and gently pulled away from the blastocyst. A laser is used to fully detach the cells from the trophectoderm (Fig. 18.2). The cells are collected and analysed using PCR- or FISH-based test.
- Blastocysts usually collapse following biopsy and are then re-examined for signs of re-expansion after further culture for up to 24 h.
- Transfer takes place when results become available, usually on day 6.

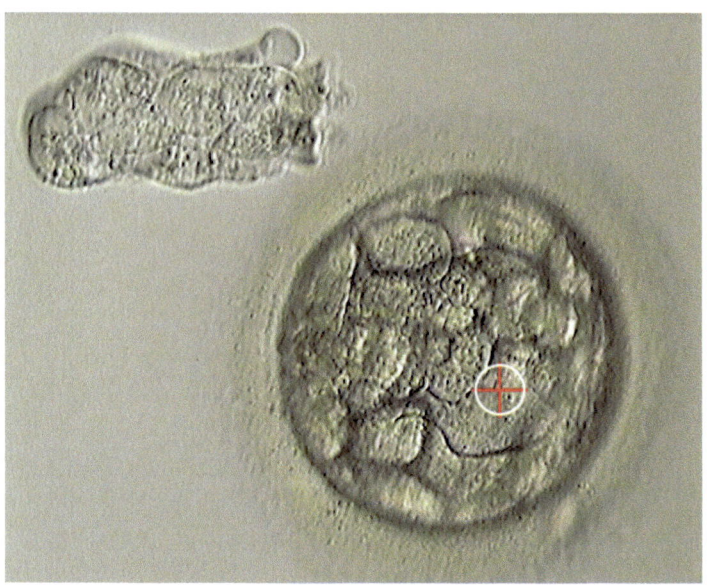

FIGURE 18.2 Blastocyst after trophectoderm biopsy, showing biopsied material

- An alternative method is to vitrify the blastocysts immediately after biopsy, before re-expansion occurs. The samples of trophectoderm can be analysed at a later date and genetically suitable embryos can be transferred in a subsequent frozen embryo transfer (FET) cycle (see Chap. 9).

As with non-PGD blastocyst culture, not all embryos will make it to the blastocyst stage, and so there may be fewer embryos available for biopsy. However, evidence suggests that live birth rates could be higher for blastocyst stage biopsy than for cleavage stage biopsy and that vitrified biopsied blastocysts have a high implantation potential when transferred in an FET cycle. This not only reduces the risk of ovarian hyperstimulation syndrome but also allows the embryos to be transferred in an FET cycle when the endometrium may be more receptive. These developments in blastocyst culture and biopsy techniques have enabled elective single blastocyst transfer to become a viable option in PGD and spare embryos to be cryopreserved for future use.

Technological Developments in PGD for Monogenic Disorders

Delivering robust tests on single cells is technically challenging due to the availability of only one copy of the genome template as the starting material. The technological field for standard diagnostic DNA testing advances quickly and new technologies are assessed to see which can be applied to PGD. Over the years, there has been a common objective of moving towards single cell tests that can be universally applied to many couples. This objective of a universal test per disease is now being replaced by the panacea of having an all-in-one test that can be applied to any couple, at risk of transmitting any genetic disease including monogenic (single gene) disorders, chromosomal translocations, HLA typing and aneuploid screening.

The majority of testing strategies for monogenic disease in preimplantation embryos use either a combination of direct mutation and linked microsatellite markers or solely linked microsatellite markers (see Chap. 8). It has been possible to implement these amplification-based tests with the availability of improved polymerases and PCR reaction mixes. It is now routine for 5 or more markers to be co-amplified and the use of 12 or more markers have been reported, thus allowing the same test to be applied to more couples. This improves the experience for couples having PGD; individualised workup is avoided and the waiting time to start a PGD cycle is reduced. Furthermore, the ability to co-amplify multiple markers can allow more than one diagnosis to be made on a single embryo such as combining a monogenic disease such as beta-thalassemia with human leukocyte antigen (HLA) typing (see Chap. 13). However, this approach still requires careful test design due to limitations in the number of markers that can be evenly co-amplified simultaneously.

Whole Genome Amplification (WGA)

As PGD involves testing only a single or, at best, few cells, more powerful and reliable amplification is required to fulfil the needs of new comprehensive whole genome studies. WGA can fulfil this need as micrograms of DNA can be produced from the 6 picograms of DNA present in a single cell for the downstream application. Various WGA systems are available. For example, WGA using isothermal amplification (non-PCR) with phi 29 DNA polymerase (REPLI-g, Qiagen; GenomiPhi, GE Healthcare) for multiple displacement amplification (MDA) produces long amplified products which are many kilobases in length and are highly representative of the starting template including accurately reproducing the number of repeat units present in a stretch of repetitive DNA sequence, the most common dinucleotide repeat being $(CA)_n$. MDA-based WGA is already used by several PGD laboratories for testing monogenic disorders as the amplified products are amenable to both genotyping and microsatellite linkage analysis.

In order to use microarrays, designed to detect copy number variation in genomic DNA, whole genome amplification of a single cell also needs to be performed. A new generation of PCR-based WGA methods is available for this purpose (SurePlex, BlueGnome; GenomePlex, Sigma-Aldrich). Following fragmentation and ligation of linker adapters to the DNA, PCR-based WGA can be performed with a turnaround time that allows array protocols to be accommodated. The genome coverage is not as representative as MDA-based WGA, due to increased amplification bias, but the accuracy is sufficient to enable detection of whole chromosome aneuploidies in single cells within a 24-h testing protocol. PCR-based WGA does not faithfully replicate microsatellite sequences; at present there is no universal WGA step for all the downstream processes required to detect both chromosome imbalance and monogenic disorders

Microarrays

Microarrays are now part of routine cytogenetic analysis for genome wide detection of copy number variations from genomic DNA. Different array platforms exist which use DNA fragments of various lengths as probes to assess copy number by comparative genomic hybridisation (aCGH). The genomic locations to be analysed are specified by the probes and these can be either cloned DNA fragments of thousands of nucleotides or synthesised DNA oligonucleotides of tens of nucleotides. At present, PCR-based WGA is the preferred method for aCGH platforms using cloned DNA probes. Clinical case reports have been reported in PGD for carriers of chromosome translocations but its main clinical use is for 24 chromosome aneuploid screening (see Chap. 16).

Single Nucleotide Polymorphism (SNP) Arrays

A SNP array is a type of oligonucleotide array which, in addition to assessing copy number, has the potential to diagnose monogenic disease by using SNP genotyping and haplotyping from family studies. The preferred method of DNA amplification for this application is MDA-WGA due to its fidelity for genotyping. Analysis of SNPs around and within the gene of interest should allow embryos to be selected based on the SNP haplotype, but as yet a clinical validation has to be completed to determine the power of this haplotyping approach over the well-established short tandem repeat (STR) microsatellite marker haplotypes. The predicted density of informative SNPs needs to be assessed for a variety of genetic scenarios including regions of high rates of recombination, telomeric or centromeric located genes, consanguinity and founder/common haplotypes.

Human Genome Sequencing

Advances in the human genome sequencing project and in single cell genomics may be of clinical use in PGD, although it was not their intended use. In PGD, parental or near relative samples are not always available for family studies in order to construct the haplotypes needed for linkage analysis. Linked markers are always used in PGD to monitor for allele dropout, contamination and recombination events and confirm any mutation result; they confer the most information when phase of the alleles is known. From the perspective of the human genome project, it is important not only to sequence but also to know on which chromosome homologue the alleles reside, since obtaining the constituent molecular haplotypes (phase defined haplotypes) of the genome will help to understand genome function (the HapMap project: hapmap.ncbi.nlm.nih.gov). It may be possible in the near future to apply metaphase chromosome isolation or other molecular haplotyping approaches from genomic projects to allow the phase of alleles to be obtained from just an individual, thus eliminating the need to seek samples from family members other than the couple requesting PGD.

Next-Generation Sequencing (NGS)

NGS has recently appeared in the repertoire of many diagnostic DNA laboratories and allows high throughput analysis of DNA by massively parallel DNA sequencing which identifies pathogenic (disease-causing) mutations in a timely and extremely cost-effective manner. The adoption by PGD centres of blastocyst biopsy and vitrification will grant the extra time needed to obtain results using NGS for genetic testing of preimplantation embryos. However, there are still technical problems to overcome. All sequencing-based strategies so far have difficulty in accurately sequencing through long repetitive DNA sequence motifs. Simple tandem repeats which include microsatellite markers and pathogenic triplet repeat mutations are likely to remain refractory to NGS analysis.

Paediatric Outcome After PGD

One of the main questions raised by the availability of PGD relates to its impact on the health and development of children born following successful treatment. Couples undertaking PGD are generally fertile and do not need assisted reproductive technology (ART) to conceive. Many parents care for children with special needs and a few have medical problems themselves as a consequence of the genetic disorder that affects them and puts their offspring at risk. Additionally, there has been a concern regarding the possible effect of embryo biopsy on the health and well-being of children born after PGD. Thus, it is important for couples wishing to have PGD to know if there is an increased risk of abnormality in the PGD babies they conceive. Therefore, follow-up of children born after PGD has been recommended since the early days of implementing PGD technology.

What Can We Learn from IVF?

IVF, with or without ICSI, has been available for over 30 years. Follow-up of infants born after IVF and ICSI has showed a relative risk of major malformation of 1.24 compared with spontaneously conceived infants. A *major malformation* is considered one that has medical or social consequences and occurs in 2–3 % of live births and 5 % of 5-year-old children. Longer-term studies have showed a relative increase risk of abnormality of 2.7 after ICSI and 1.8 after IVF. An increase in imprinting disorders such as Beckwith-Wiedemann (BWS) and Angelman syndromes and retinoblastoma has also been reported in IVF/ICSI babies.

PGD Neonatal Data

Studies reporting on the abnormality rate detected in children after PGD comprise single-centre studies and studies based on international databases such as the ESHRE PGD

Consortium database (see Chap. 11). Typically, single-centre studies include the evaluation of hundreds of PGD babies, whilst international databases report on thousands of babies born after PGD. Recent data from the various studies suggest that the major abnormality rate at birth after PGD ranges from 1.6 to 2.1 %. Some babies have more than 1 abnormality. The abnormalities ranged from significant cardiac abnormalities to mild syndactyly. These outcomes are comparable to those reported in the IVF/ICSI population.

In addition, no differences were found in the incidence of preterm birth, neonatal weight, length and head circumference between PGD babies and babies born after IVF/ICSI. Likewise, the perinatal mortality rates after PGD and IVF/ICSI were comparable. No data exists comparing the rate of birth defects in PGD infants with naturally conceived infants.

Later Outcome Studies

In our centre, we followed up 120 PGD babies born between 1999 and 2007. Data about health and development was collated at birth and 1 and 2 years of age. At birth, seven babies were found to have minor or major malformations. By 2 years of age, few new abnormalities were reported, leaving us to conclude that longer-term follow-up of PGD infants was necessary. A few studies have investigated long-term development of children born following PGD, although such data remains limited and typically involves up to 100 children only in each study. Those studies reported that PGD children were of lower birth weight, but their linear growth and incidence of childhood ill health was comparable to that of normally conceived children. In addition, mental and psychomotor development at 2 years of age was also found to be similar to the control groups, as was social, emotional and language development.

Factors That Could Influence Birth Outcome

- Maternal age and parity
- Maternal health

- Pre-pregnancy maternal body mass index
- Multiple pregnancy
- Duration of gestation
- Environmental factors, e.g., smoking and alcohol consumption

Recommendations for Paediatric Follow-Up of PGD Babies

- As the number of PGD babies born remains small, international collaboration and routine standardised data collection is required for effective long-term follow-up.
- Couples need to be made aware of the additional, albeit small, risk of abnormality associated with treatment prior to undergoing PGD.
- Any woman who has health-related problems associated with the genetic diagnosis should be referred to an obstetric or other relevant physician to discuss the optimum management of her condition during pregnancy and labour.
- Every effort should be made to minimise the risk of multiple birth after PGD treatment.

Key Points
- Trophectoderm biopsy for PGD provides a larger DNA sample for robust genetic testing and could be associated with improved PGD outcome.
- A universal all-in-one PGD test is a realistic objective, but further development of molecular testing technology is required.
- Large co-ordinated international paediatric follow-up studies are needed to confirm long term safety of PGD.
- Efforts should be made to minimise the risk of multiple births after PGD.

Further Reading

Chang LJ, Huang CC, Tsai YY, Hung CC, Fang MY, Lin YC, Su YN, Chen SU, Yang YS. Blastocyst biopsy and vitrification are effective for preimplantation genetic diagnosis of monogenic diseases. Hum Reprod. 2013;28(5):1435–44.

Desmyttere S, De Rycke M, Staessen C, Liebaers I, De Schrijver F, Verpoest W, Haentjens P, Boundelle M. Neonatal follow-up of 995 consecutively born children after embryo biopsy for PGD. Hum Reprod. 2012;27:288–93.

Fan H, Wang J, Potanina A, Quake SR. Whole genome molecular haplotyping of single cells. Nat Biotechnol. 2011;29(1):51–7.

Handyside A, Harton GL, Mariani B, Thornhill AR, Affara N, Shaw MA, Griffin DK. Karyomapping: a universal method for genome wide analysis of genetic disease based on mapping crossovers between parental haplotypes. J Med Genet. 2010;47(10):651–8.

Harper JC, Wilton L, Traeger-Synodinos J, Goossens V, Moutou C, SenGupta SB, Pehlivan Budak T, Renwick P, De Rycke M, Geraedts JP, Harton G. The ESHRE PGD consortium: 10 years of data collection. Hum Reprod Update. 2012;18(3):234–47.

Hosomichi K, Jinam TA, Mitsunaga S, Nakaoka H, Inoue I. Phase determined complete sequencing of the HLA genes by next generation sequencing. BMC Genomics. 2013;14:355–70.

Lashwood A, Kanabar D, El-Toukhy T, Kavalier F. Paediatric outcome from birth onwards after preimplantation genetic diagnosis. J Med Genet. 2007;44 Suppl 1:S28.

Liebaers I, Desmyttere S, Verpoest W, De Rycke M, Staessen C, Sermon K, Devroey P, Haentjens P, Bonduelle M. Report on a consecutive series of 581 children born after blastomere biopsy for preimplantation genetic diagnosis. Hum Reprod. 2010;25(1):275–82.

Lim D, Bowdin SC, Tee L, Kirby GA, Blair E, Fryer A, Lam W, Oley C, Cole T, Brueton LA, Reik W, Macdonald F, Maher ER. Clinical and molecular genetic features of Beckwith-Wiedemann syndrome associated with assisted reproductive technologies. Hum Reprod. 2009;24(3):741–7.

Nekkebroeck J, Bonduelle M, Desmyttere S, Van den Broeck W, Ponjaert-Kristoffersen I. Mental and psychomotor development of 2-year-old children born after preimplantation genetic diagnosis/screening. Hum Reprod. 2008;23:1560–6.

Nekkebroeck J, Bonduelle M, Desmyttere S, Van den Broeck W, Ponjaert-Kristoffersen I. Socioemotional and language development of 2-year-old children born after PGD/PGS, and parental well-being. Hum Reprod. 2008;23:1849–57.

Thornhill AR, DeDie-Smulders CE, Geraedts JP, Harper JC, Harton GL, Lavery SA, et al. ESHRE PGD consortium. ESHRE PGD consortium 'best practice guidelines for clinical preimplantation genetic diagnosis (PGD) and preimplantation genetic screening (PGS)'. Hum Reprod. 2005;20:35–48.

Treff NR, Fedick A, Tao X, Devkota B, Taylor D, Scott Jr RT. Evaluation of targeted next-generation sequencing-based preimplantation genetic diagnosis of monogenic disease. Fertil Steril. 2013;99(5):1377–84.

Xu K, Montag M. New perspectives on embryo biopsy: not how, but when and why? Semin Reprod Med. 2012;30(4):259–66.

Chapter 19
The Future of Preimplantation Genetic Testing: From Research Lab to Responsible Patient Care

Peter Braude and Caroline Mackie Ogilvie

Our understanding of the genetics and biology of the early developing human has improved with the drive for better ways to deliver preimplantation testing clinically. Susceptibility to human aneuploidy during meiosis has been confirmed and the ubiquity of post zygotic mosaicism has been revealed by the research on embryos aimed to test the validity of diagnosis from single-cell biopsy.

The clinical need for PGD is to select embryos free from a familial mutation, free from chromosome imbalance consequent on a parental chromosome rearrangement, or to select embryos free from aneuploidy in order to improve IVF success rates. Previous chapters in this book describe the theory

P. Braude, MB, BCh, PhD, FRCOG, FMedSci, FSB (✉)
Division of Women's Health, King's College London,
St. Thomas' Hospital, Westminster Bridge Road,
London SE1 7EH, UK
e-mail: peter.braude@kcl.ac.uk

C.M. Ogilvie, BSc, DPhil
Cytogenetics Department, Guy's and St. Thomas' NHS Foundation Trust, 5th Floor, Tower Wing, London SE1 9RT, UK
e-mail: caroline.ogilvie@genetics.kcl.ac.uk

T. El-Toukhy, P. Braude (eds.), *Preimplantation Genetic Diagnosis in Clinical Practice*, DOI 10.1007/978-1-4471-2948-6_19,
© Springer-Verlag London 2014

of PGD and the standard, validated protocols. This chapter examines future possibilities for preimplantation genetic testing.

Progress and improvements in preimplantation genetic testing historically have been driven by technological advance; for instance, FISH probes for the ends of chromosomes, methods for the faithful amplification of the whole genome from a single cell and the development of array technology have, respectively, allowed PGD for chromosome rearrangements, preimplantation genetic haplotyping and the screening of embryo biopsies across all the chromosomes for detection of aneuploidy. Likewise, the rapid recent advances in the development of further cheap, efficient and accurate techniques for interrogating the human genome are opening new possibilities for preimplantation testing. Coincident with advances in testing methods, there have been huge leaps in molecular biology techniques allowing more and more information to be gathered on limited samples of material, and progress in automation, robotics and computation has facilitated the ability to test more samples more quickly and at yearly decreasing costs.

Recent methods relevant to PGD include qPCR and array technologies, such as array CGH, SNP arrays and karyomapping (Chap. 18) which are already being used in PGD for the detection of aneuploidy and unbalanced products of parental chromosome rearrangements. However, additional imbalances *within* chromosomes (i.e. deletion or duplication of genetic material) also can be detected. These changes known as copy number variants (CNVs) may be benign or pathogenic, depending on their size and gene content. Postnatal testing of control populations using arrays has shown that most individuals carry CNVs, many of them *private* family CNVs; interpreting the clinical significance of a previously undescribed CNV therefore can be problematic, particularly in the context of prenatal or preimplantation testing.

Perhaps the most dramatic recent advance in genome technology has been the development of next generation sequencing (NGS). It took around 10 years and a cost of

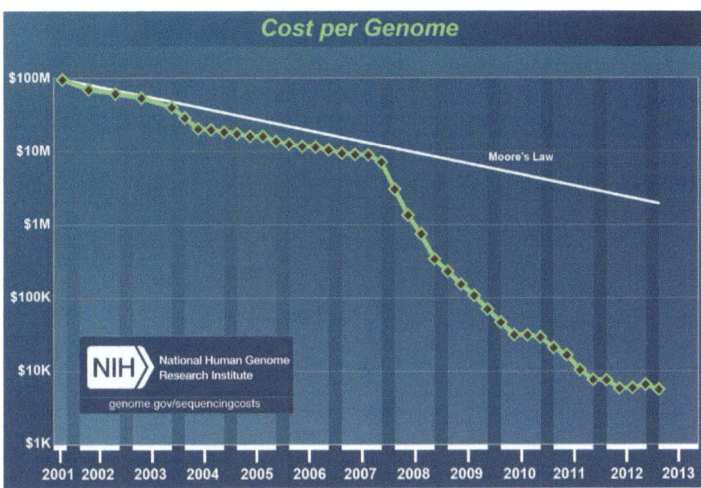

FIGURE. 19.1 'Cost per Genome' — the cost of sequencing a human-sized genome (Wetterstrand KA. DNA sequencing costs: data from the NHGRI genome sequencing program (GSP). Available at: www.genome.gov/sequencingcosts. Courtesy: National Human Genome Research Institute: www.genome.gov)

many millions of dollars to complete the first sequence of the human genome using 'Sanger' sequencing, but using the latest semiconductor technology, it is now possible to sequence an entire genome in a day, for a cost of around $1,000, although the accuracy of this technique is yet to be established (Fig. 19.1). The continuing development of cheaper and more efficient methods for NGS has led to suggestions that this technology could be used for PGD, giving genome-wide information on mutations.

The potential for providing such detailed genome-wide information raises particular practical, clinical and ethical problems not previously considered as part of preimplantation testing. As with CNV detection, the significance of any mutations detected may be unknown, providing dilemmas for the selection of embryos for transfer. Further understanding of the human genome by collecting information postnatally on common polymorphisms and variants of currently unknown significance will be needed before NGS can be applied confidently to PGD in the clinic. In addition, a patient who seeks PGD will have had extensive counselling for the particular disease that they are seeking to avoid and have discussed the practicalities of the test including misdiagnosis, non-diagnosis and the possibility of having few or no embryos to replace after testing. The appearance of a different disease-causing mutation at another site may not only have consequences for the individual but might have consequences for other siblings and members of the extended family. For example, the finding of a haemophilia mutation in an embryo being tested for cystic fibrosis might have consequences for other male children in the family and other male children of relatives. Furthermore, the fact that an additional disease-causing mutation has been detected potentially reduces the cohort of disease-free embryos available from that cycle.

Since a multitude of disease-causing mutations could be identified using these techniques, including those which for practical reasons could not be covered even in a comprehensive counselling session, it raises the question as to whether the information at these sites should be revealed or whether they should be left unexamined and thus left 'undiscovered'. There are consequences both ways: by revealing the information, anxiety is caused, and embryos excluded from transfer, thus drastically reducing the cohort of available embryos; concealing a mutation which could result in disability would be inexcusable, and not examining for potentially helpful and life-saving information could be regarded as negligent.

It should be appreciated that, apart from new mutations generated during formation of sperm and eggs, and the development of the embryo, the genetic information that could be revealed following detailed genetic testing of the embryo is already present in the parents and thus could be tested pre-conceptually. Use of preconception screening of the parents for mutations in genes known to be associated with recessive disease, agreed mutually between clinician and the couple, would substantially diminish the likelihood of surprises. It may be possible to draw up protocols for obtaining patient consent for examining only these loci, and others where mutations cause known pathology of complete penetrance. However, there is inherent uncertainty of secure diagnosis using limited cells taken from a restricted part of the embryo, and the more mutations that are examined, the less likely it is that there will be any embryos left for transfer. Whether the full set of information should be kept for the child's later use as part of its medical history is open to debate, as advances in sequencing technology are likely to make information from current techniques redundant by the time the child has need of it.

These evolving methods still take time to execute, and depending on the technology used, it may not be possible to biopsy a blastocyst and have the result ready in time for a same-day transfer. Biopsy at the cleavage stage would allow more time but decreases accuracy of diagnosis due to mosaicism and paucity of material. Improvements in cryopreservation now allow dislocation of biopsy and DNA extraction from the diagnostic test. Blastocysts can be biopsied and vitrified and stored pending the diagnostic result. Transfer can then be undertaken as a subsequent elective procedure. Although predicated on effective cryostorage and thawing, this method probably holds more advantages than disadvantages. The biopsied material can be stored, allowing the diagnostic tests to be batched and tested electively. This means that:

- Any unexpected findings can be discussed with the patient without the pressure of transfer looming, allowing them time to consider their choices and for further genetic counselling.
- Frozen embryo transfer can be scheduled for patient convenience and in a natural cycle, which may be more conducive to implantation and healthy babies.
- The pressure on achieving a genetic result in a limited time frame is relieved, and there is more time to evaluate and interpret the results.

- More cases can be undertaken on 1 day and be distributed more easily during the week, avoiding weekend working if needed.
- Critically, it also facilitates the transfer of a single embryo, thus reducing the chance of multiple pregnancies. Should pregnancy not follow, additional scheduled transfers can take place if there are more frozen embryos available.

Will the Promise of New Technology Necessarily Deliver Better Results?

Numerous claims of efficacy for preimplantation genetic testing have been made over the years, but a number have failed due to inadequate structured clinical research prior to formal clinical implementation. Preimplantation genetic screening (PGS) is offered in many countries as a form of PGD and is numerically the largest reason given for embryo biopsy. At least ten randomised clinical trials have now shown that FISH on single blastomeres removed at cleavage stage is ineffective, as it does not improve delivery rates after IVF (Chap. 16). Not only is FISH diagnosis limited by the number of probes that can be used simultaneously or sequentially, and hence not all chromosomes can be tested for, but mosaicism between blastomeres can lead to false positive and false negative results as biopsies may not be representative of the genetic status of the whole embryo. The reasons for this particular fiasco endure and provide important learning points for implementation of new genetic techniques to PGD in the future: enthusiasm and belief over sound evidence; premature clinical implementation driven by media hype, unrealistic patient expectations and commercial pressure; and failure to understand the biology of the early embryo. Another important point regarding the use of NGS for diagnosis is that DNA sequence is not the sole determinant of phenotypic outcome. Epigenetics plays a crucial role in regulating gene activity and there is as yet no clinically applicable genome-wide test for disturbances in epigenetic marking. Selection of an embryo with no deleterious mutations is therefore not a guarantee of a disease-free child.

We are once more entering a period where expectations are high and where preliminary results are being offered as a sure panacea. Patients unfulfilled by the failures of previous methods are pinning their hopes on improvements to technology. Sadly, the biology is unchanged and our understanding still limited. The evidence to say that blastocysts have sufficiently low mosaicism for a test to be reliable is scant, and we have no idea how cells with differing genetic make-up are distributed as the embryo develops. There are suggestions that embryos with significant mosaicism of aneuploidy even at the morula stage are able to self-correct and hence would be discarded unnecessarily on inappropriate testing. Whether the use of array CGH, through which the full chromosome set can be examined, and whether its use on more cells which can easily be biopsied from the trophectoderm at the blastocyst stage will improve PGS outcome is yet to be demonstrated in appropriately structured clinical trials.

What Do Patients Want from Preimplantation Testing and How Is This Likely to Be Delivered in the Future?

Patients who have a family history of genetic disease, or who have given birth to a child with disability as a result, are keen to try and avoid a recurrence. As outlined in Chap. 2, there are a number of ways of achieving this, only one of which is PGD. Many couples will still opt for prenatal diagnosis but are concerned at the gestation at which it is usually performed and the significant development of the fetus before they may have to consider termination of the pregnancy. There is an increasing expectation that new tests for free fetal DNA circulating in the maternal circulation might lower the time at which a diagnosis could be made and hence allow for very early termination.

This test requires distinguishing unequivocally the tiny amounts of early fetal DNA from the huge sea of free DNA and cells present in the mother's circulation, an extraordinarily complex task. Current techniques are only sufficiently sensitive to make this distinction from about 11 weeks gestation thus conferring little advantage in diagnostic time, other than avoiding invasive prenatal procedures. Unless there are significant technical advances in the future that allow smaller amounts of DNA to be distinguished reliably and hence at earlier stages, it is likely that PGD will remain the preferred option.

Should We Choose Our Children? Use of Positive Selection

Since the introduction of prenatal diagnosis and subsequently PGD, there have been concerns that emerging genetic technologies will be used for eugenic purposes. These concerns have been exacerbated by the immense power of molecular methods especially as applied to embryos. There is concern that the ability to reveal very detailed information about the personal genome will provide opportunities for extensive embryo selection for non-medical reasons.

Whilst there are proponents of a moral obligation to create children with the chance of the best life (procreative beneficence), the opposing view of the child as a gift with an acceptance of that child's talents or disabilities is more usual. The use of PGD falls somewhere in between; where severe disability or life-threatening illness can be avoided in order to provide a better life, it should be allowed to be used. Nevertheless, it is clear that if untargeted diagnosis is performed, information could be revealed that would allow more choice, albeit limited by the parental genetic make-up. Even with current technology, sex selection is possible not only by PGD but also by selecting for X- or Y-bearing sperm. Indeed, a 2008 survey of 190 US clinics showed that 42 % would provide PGD for medical conditions but would also select embryos with the patients' preferred gender. In an unregulated market, it is unclear how far patients would go in the pursuit of additional traits to that being tested for by PGD and how compliant clinics and clinicians would be. In the UK, the presence of a regulator (the HFEA) operating under well-established law (HFE Act 1991 and 2008) restricts sex selection to medical need and precludes testing that deliberately enhances the chance of genetic mutation. Licences are needed for each type of disease being tested for, and a code of practice limits the use of PGS.

It is likely that as the cost of these technologies continues to fall, similar debates to those held at the inception of PGD will begin. The challenge for those working in this field will surely be to apply these new methodologies wisely, in the best interests of patients, and to avoid the temptation to be swept along on a tide of innovative technology. And it is important to remember that however sophisticated the available technology, the opportunities for embryo selection will always be constrained by the parental gene pool and the limited size of embryo cohort, at least until gene modification becomes technically possible and ethically approved.

Key Points
- Progress and improvements in preimplantation genetic testing historically have been driven by technological advance. Powerful new genetic technologies are being applied to PGT before their nuances or consequences are fully understood.
- We are once more entering a period where expectations are high and where preliminary results are being offered as a sure panacea. Patients unfulfilled by the failures of previous methods are pinning their hopes on improvements to technology and being offered new tests prior to demonstration of their efficacy by appropriately structured clinical trials.

- The potential for discovering genome-wide information by techniques such as next generation sequencing raises particular practical, clinical and ethical problems not previously considered as part of preimplantation testing.
- As most genetic information that could be revealed following detailed genetic testing of the embryo is already present in the parents, the use of preconception screening of the parents for mutations known to be associated with recessive disease would substantially diminish the likelihood of genetic surprises.
- Since the introduction of prenatal diagnosis and subsequently PGD, there have been concerns that emerging genetic technologies will be used for eugenic purposes. There is again concern that the ability to reveal very detailed information about the personal genome could provide opportunities for extensive embryo selection for non-medical reasons.

Recommended Reading and Resources

de Jong A, Dondorp WJ, Frints SGM, de Die-Smulders CEM, de Wert GMWR. Advances in prenatal screening: the ethical dimension. Nat Rev Genet. 2011;12:657–63.

DNA sequencing costs. Data from the NHGRI genome sequencing program (GSP). http://www.genome.gov/sequencingcosts/.

Fragouli E, Wells D. Aneuploidy in the human blastocyst. Cytogenet Genome Res. 2011;133:149–59.

Handyside A. PGD and aneuploidy screening for 24 chromosomes by genome-wide SNP analysis: seeing the wood and the trees. Reprod Biomed Online. 2011;23:686–91.

https://notendur.hi.is/~sigma/PDFfiles/Savulescu.pdf.

Human Fertilisation and Embryology Authority. Review of sex selection. 2002. http://www.hfea.gov.uk/517.html.

Julian S, Guy K. The moral obligation to create children with the best chance of the best life. Bioethics. 2009;23(5):274–90.

Sandel MJ. The case against perfection. The Atlantic Monthly. Apr 2004. http://jrichardstevens.com/articles/sandel-genetics.pdf.

Savulescu J. Procreative beneficence: why we should select the best children. Bioethics. 2001;15(5/6):413–26.

The Human Genome Project; Wellcome Trust Sanger Institute. http://www.sanger.ac.uk/about/history/hgp/.

Index

T. El-Toukhy, P. Braude (eds.), *Preimplantation Genetic
Diagnosis in Clinical Practice*, DOI 10.1007/978-1-4471-2948-6,
© Springer-Verlag London 2014